Foundations in Nursing and Health Care

Introduction to Research

Mark Walsh and Lynne Wigens
Series Editor: Lynne Wigens

T

Text © Mark Walsh and Lynne Wigens 2003
Original illustrations © Nelson Thornes Ltd 2003

Published in 2003 by:
Nelson Thornes Ltd
Delta Place
27 Bath Road
CHELTENHAM
GL53 7TH
United Kingdom

05 06 07 / 10 9 8 7 6 5 4 3 2

A catalogue record for this book is available from the British Library

ISBN 0 7487 7118 2

Illustrations by Clinton Banbury
Page make-up by Michael Fay

Printed in Croatia by Zrinski

Contents

Acknowledgements

The authors would like to thank Helen Broadfield from Nelson Thornes for her guidance during the development of this book.

Special thanks from Mark Walsh to Karen Seymour for her love and support, and from Lynne Wigens to Paul, Matthew and Samuel for their support and encouragement.

Introduction

This book has been written for people who are new to research and are faced with the prospect of having to critically read research papers or carry out a small-scale research investigation. In particular, the book aims to help students who are commencing the first year of a health-care course such as nursing, midwifery, physiotherapy or occupational therapy. As well as covering general principles and approaches to research, the book can also act as a guide to the process of actually doing a piece of practical research.

While writing the book we have tried to take into account the situation and pressures that are typically faced by students on health-care courses. In particular, we are aware that many students are required to read research articles and do a small-scale research project early on in their course. However, understanding research study is only part of what readers have to do alongside their other clinical work, study and personal life commitments. As such, the book aims to help readers to control and manage their learning about research, so that it does not absorb too much time or get out of hand.

The book has been put together in a way that gives guidance, support and ideas in the areas where first-year students tend to need them. We have learnt about this during many years of teaching research methods and supervising student researchers on health and social courses. The more understanding you have of how research investigation works the less daunting the prospect of 'doing research' becomes. In fact, some students go as far as describing doing a small research project as a fantastic and thrilling experience.

Knowledge and understanding of research methods is important in many professions and areas of life. Doing your first project will help you to gain an insight into what 'research' can mean, and it will help you to think critically about the strengths and weaknesses of reported research in the future.

Structure of the book

The book is divided into 13 chapters.

The first four chapters are designed to give you an introduction and explanation of the basic purpose of research. Knowledge and understanding of research investigation is helped by looking at what makes research investigation different from some other forms of information-seeking and the importance of research to health care. In Chapter 3, we will be taking a closer look at the ideas and assumptions underpinning two key theoretical approaches to research investigation. The choice that is made about which approach is adopted has a big effect on how a research investigation develops. The links between research, evidence-based practice and clinical audit are explained. These early chapters 'set the scene' by explaining the stages in the research process. The importance of doing a lot of your thinking and planning before any data is collected can not be over-emphasised. Careful preparation is a strategy for success in research. One of the lessons of small-scale projects learned by many first-time researchers is that they should have invested more time and effort in their preparation.

The next four chapters (Chapters 5–8) focus on reading research reports and background literature effectively. Although reading research could be the final goal for many health-care practitioners, it may also be the starting point for deciding on an area for possible investigation. We will explore the practicalities of developing a research question in Chapter 6.

The final five chapters of the book (Chapters 9–13) focus on the practicalities of collecting and analysing data and then producing a research report. Actually getting research data is much less difficult than making sense of it. Throughout the text examples of research articles using particular research strategies and methods are given. A whole chapter (Chapter 11) is given over to ethical considerations in research, as this is particularly important in the health-care field. Chapter 13 stresses how all the decisions that you will have made while following a research process are 'pulled together', described and explained in your research report. The chapter explains what readers expect to see when they open a research report. Overall, the structure of the book follows a step-by-step approach that could help you to get from the beginning to the end of a small-scale project.

The book is structured to take you from being a complete novice regarding research to an evaluator of research and an informed small-scale researcher. Some readers may work through it section by section, while others may prefer to dip in and out of it as they require information. The book is flexible enough to meet various needs and will contribute positively to the successful completion of your health-care course.

1

Research and its role in health care

Learning outcomes

By the end of this chapter you should be able to:

● Define what research is and the key characteristics of research

● Identify the stages of the research process

What is a research investigation?

Textbooks usually adopt one of two main approaches to defining what 'research' is. The first approach sees research as a range of practical skills and activities that are used to conduct particular types of investigation. This approach defines research in terms of what researchers do and the ways in which they do it. A second approach sees research as a way of thinking (Kumar 1996). In this approach, research is about asking critical questions, thinking about and examining evidence and using this to understand phenomena, issues or problems more clearly.

Both these approaches are useful ways of understanding and defining what is involved in a research investigation. As a result, a third approach is to say that a research investigation involves both a particular way of thinking and an identifiable range of skills and activities. Within this book we are going to cover both the practical skills and activities and the thinking part of doing a research investigation. We will also look at how to understand other peoples' research and use it in health-care settings.

Characteristics of research investigations

It is important at this early stage that you see a research investigation as something more than asking a group of people a few questions or looking up a topic in several books and then summarising your findings. You have probably heard of people doing this and saying that they have done some research. Real research investigations involve more than this kind of general seeking of information. The types of research investigation that you are going to learn about involve:

● Putting forward ideas that can be *tested*

● Collecting data to test these ideas in a *systematic* way

● *Analysing* the collected data

● Drawing conclusions based on the research *evidence*

According to Kumar (1996), research investigations should follow a **process** that:

- Is undertaken within a clear philosophical framework
- Uses procedures, methods and techniques that are evaluated for their *validity* and *reliability*
- Is designed to be *unbiased* and *objective*.

The term **research process** is very important here. A process is a series of actions or an accepted method of doing something. While research investigation is exciting because it is about discovering and exploring, professional and academic researchers tend to go about their discovering and exploring in a controlled, rigorous and systematic way. In other words, they follow a research process.

Following a research process

A research process is simply a planned, structured approach to inquiry that ensures that your investigation proceeds in a logical, coherent way. There is no one perfect way to conduct a research investigation, so there is no single model of the research process as such. There is, however, a broadly accepted series of phases that should be a part of a process of research inquiry.

Researchers have to complete a number of different activities as they work through each phase of their research process. Within the text and activities outlined in the remaining chapters of the book the issues and decisions that researchers face are discussed.

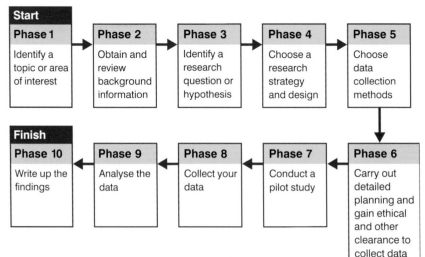

Figure 1.1 *A 10-phase version of the research process*

○━π *Keywords*

Ontological

Ontological assumptions are the researcher's views about the nature of reality

Epistemological

Epistemological assumptions are the researcher's decisions about how best to gather research data on this reality

Why bother to do research investigations?

Knowledge produced through research investigation is generally valued more highly than, and can be contrasted with, a common-sense or opinion-based understanding of the world. Common sense is based on unquestioned, taken-for-granted assumptions, while opinions reflect personal prejudices, preferences and ideals. Research-based knowledge, on the other hand, is based on *empirical evidence*, i.e. scientific evidence that comes from observation and experience of the real world.

How do you know what you know?

Research evidence is a form of knowledge that is typically based on a 'scientific' way of viewing reality or the 'truth' about the world. Health-care workers need to make judgements about what is correct or true in an endless variety of situations that affect their clinical practice. Have you ever wondered how you do this? You may not always consciously think about the basis of your decision making but whenever you do make a clinical decision you are drawing on some form of knowledge.

Epistemology is the theory of knowledge, it is:

concerned with how we know what we know, what justifies us believing what we do, and what standards of evidence we should use in seeking truths about the world and human experience.

Audi 1998, p. 1

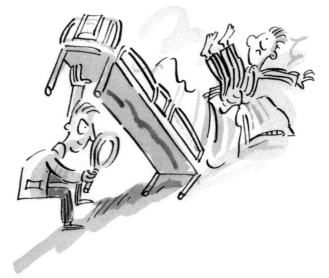

Many researchers believe that The Truth is out there and it's their job to find it

Health-care knowledge is predominantly empirical or scientific in nature, but other forms of knowledge are also important in understanding health-care practice. For instance, the forms of knowledge that influence a decision to withdraw active treatment for a patient with cancer are not simply based on research data. Personal beliefs (cultural and religious, for example) as well as subjective judgements about pain and quality of life are also likely to be part of the 'knowledge' that underpins this type of decision.

Carper (1978) identifies four ways of knowing about health-care practice:

1. Empirical: scientific knowledge
2. Aesthetic: the art of performing practical skills through experience
3. Personal: the way health-care staff view and use themselves
4. Ethical: practice dilemmas and making moral decisions.

Despite the obvious importance of empirical or scientific knowledge to health care, the other forms of knowing identified by Carper (1978) show that more than one epistemological approach is needed if the true diversity of good practice is to occur.

Why use research-based knowledge in health care?

There are lots of situations in which common sense and opinions are not a good enough basis for making decisions or developing understanding. For example, research can provide objective evidence that assists health and social policy-makers in deciding on ways of addressing issues or apparent problems in a local community.

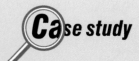

Case study

Meera's research study

Meera is a community nurse with special responsibility for issues related to sexual health and pregnancy. She is concerned that the teenage pregnancy rate in her town is relatively high compared to other areas around the UK. The view of many local people is that girls who get pregnant do so deliberately, to gain housing from the council, and that the problem of teenage pregnancy is the result of some girls' bad parenting and poor upbringing. Meera believes that this common-sense, opinion-based explanation of teenage pregnancy is unsatisfactory. She thinks that a sexual health promotion strategy for teenagers should be based on empirical evidence about local teenagers' knowledge and attitudes towards sex, contraception and relationships. Meera's intended research study will look at the sexual health knowledge, attitudes and behaviour of male and female teenagers in her local area. She feels that her research findings will provide an objective basis on which to plan her health promotion strategy.

Researchers generally aim to produce knowledge that is useful and that extends human understanding. The findings of research investigations can, at one extreme, lead to new theories that extend knowledge in disciplines such as health, social care and the social sciences. Other types of research investigation can also produce practically useful findings that influence and help policy-makers and practitioners working in fields such as health, welfare and education.

RRRRRRapid recap

Check your progress so far by working through each of the following questions.
1. Give three terms that describe research and indicate the difference between research and other forms of knowledge.
2. Explain what the term 'epistemology' means.
3. Jot down the different stages of the research process.

If you have difficulty with more than one of the questions, read through the section again to refresh your understanding before moving on.

References

Audi, R. (1998) *Epistemology: A contemporary introduction to the theory of knowledge*. Routledge, London.

Carper, B. (1978) Fundamental patterns of knowing in nursing. *Advances in Nursing Sciences*, **1**, 13–23.

Kumar, R. (1996) *Research Methodology*. Sage Publications, London.

Further reading

Benner, P. (1984) *From Novice to Expert: Excellence and power in clinical nursing practice*. Addison-Wesley, Menlo Park, CA.

Bird, S., Nicholls, G. and White, E. (1995) An overview of the research methodologies available to the occupational therapist and an outline of the research process. *British Journal of Occupational Therapy*, **58**, 510–516.

Green, S. (2000) *Research Methods in Health, Social and Early Years Care*. Stanley Thornes, Cheltenham, pp. 1–11.

2 Linking research to evidence-based practice and audit

Learning outcomes

By the end of this chapter you should be able to:

- Define evidence-based practice and the stages of implementation of evidence-based practice
- Discriminate between audit, research and evidence-based practice

What forms of knowledge influence practice?

There is an increasing emphasis on research in health care. *Clinical governance* is the term that encompasses everything that helps to maintain and improve the standards and delivery of health care to patients. Clinical governance includes:

- **Clinical audit**: monitoring of existing practice and improvements to this
- **Clinical risk management**: recognising, acting and learning from mistakes or poor performance
- **Quality assurance**: quality-monitoring processes
- **Staff development**: training, education and skills development
- **Clinical effectiveness**: promoting improvements and good practice.

Clinical effectiveness is the extent to which clinical interventions, when used for a particular patient, or population, do what they are intended to do (NHS Executive 1996). To show that their practice is clinically effective, health-care professionals need to obtain and implement evidence of this, evaluate the impact of the changed practice and show that they have contributed to better patient outcomes.

When you make a clinical decision as a health-care professional, different forms of knowledge can be involved, including:

- Past experience
- Trial and error
- Authority (e.g. hospital policy)
- Traditional custom and practice
- Clinical intuition
- Research.

tɔɘ̀ʟɘЯ Rɘ̀ʟʟɘɔ**Reflective activity**

Why do you do what you do?

Reflect on an action you recently took with a patient. What did you do?
Your action could have been to explain a medical intervention, e.g. surgery.
What was the *underlying reason* that you took the approach you did?
Perhaps you sat down with the patient and discussed the surgery, and to do
this you might have used an information leaflet that included diagrams.
Whatever action you have chosen to reflect on, you need to decide why you
chose the approach you did rather than some other approach.

Evaluating possible 'sources of knowledge'

In the example given, a nurse might decide to use an information
leaflet combined with a verbal discussion because from past
experience they have come to see that patients understand and cope
better with surgery when they have it explained in this way. Various
ways of explaining the surgery, including videos or models, may have
been tried previously, and through 'trial and error' it may have been
determined that verbal discussion backed up with an information
leaflet was the 'best' approach. It may be that the nurse was just
following the surgical ward's policy in preoperative information-giving,
or that, as a result of tradition and watching others, the nurse has
always done it in this way. Perhaps the way the nurse gave the
preoperative information was based on what they felt intuitively
would work with a particular patient. Or it may be that the nurse
was aware of a research study showing that the combination of verbal
and written preoperative information leads to increased retention of
the information and that patients informed in this way experience
significantly less anxiety.

Each of these underlying reasons represent a 'source of knowledge'
used to make a clinical decision. In undertaking the last activity
you should have identified the basis of your clinical reasoning.
Was your action based on research? The risk, if it was not, is that
not all sources of knowledge are highly reliable and, when applied,
they may not consistently produce desired patient outcomes.

Theory and **Practice**

Two useful questions to ask yourself each year as you increase in health care experience are:

● How much of your clinical practice is knowingly based on research?

● How many times have you changed your practice due to new evidence becoming available?

What is evidence-based practice?

Recently there has been a movement towards 'evidence-based practice' in health care. Evidence-based health care involves the 'conscientious, explicit and judicious use of current best evidence about the care of individual patients' (Sackett *et al.* 1996, p. 71).

This often-quoted definition suggests that, in order to approach your care in an 'evidence-based' way, you need to review the evidence available, thinking carefully and clearly about what makes most sense in influencing your clinical decisions. The 'best' part of the definition means that, wherever possible, scientific research that is relevant and properly conducted should be used. Evidence-based practice also means integrating individual clinical expertise with the best available external evidence.

There are advantages for health-care professionals who practise in an evidence-based way as it means that their knowledge base continues to improve and that they have increased confidence in their clinical decision-making. Busy health-care professionals want to use research but can find it difficult to find the time to keep abreast of advances in practice through reading journals and other external evidence, let alone undertaking their own research studies.

Research needs to be relevant to the clinical situation, acceptable to the professional and the patient, comprehensive, accurate, easily accessible and understandable if nurses and other health-care professionals are to implement the findings. We are most familiar with original research studies that, for instance, compare two different hand-washing methods. It is very rare for a single research study to offer a final, irrefutable answer to a clinical question.

In addition, you may find that two studies that look at the same clinical question give very different answers. This may be due to differences in the research process. Study A may conclude that the two versions of hand-washing show no difference in the degree to which they reduce levels of bacteria, whereas study B may suggest that one form of hand-washing significantly reduces the level of bacteria in comparison to the other. In this example, the conflicting evidence would be an inadequate base for a decision on hand-washing practices for the clinical area. For this reason, the evidence-based practice movement has led to the combining of research evidence from a number of studies, including ranking of the strength, level and validity of the evidence. How different forms of research are compared is examined below in the section 'How is research to be judged?'

How do you implement evidence-based practice?

Evidence-based practice is a total process (Figure 2.1) beginning with knowing what clinical questions to ask.

First, you need to identify an area of practice for which the evidence base is not known. Then you need to search for relevant literature using a range of sources, such as libraries, electronic databases on the Internet and colleagues. If systematic reviews (summaries of all the available research in an area) already exist, you should use these.

Once all the relevant literature has been read and critically examined (see Chapter 8 for ways of critiquing research) you should share this information with other staff to find out whether they think it is relevant to practice. A comparison needs to be made between the 'best practice' you have identified through the literature search and the practice that currently exists. The question then needs to be asked as to whether a change in practice is needed. The evidence you have found may now support your previously unsupported practice, or you may need to manage a change in practice.

The next stage will be to implement the findings of your evidence-based practice review into your practice area. 'Old habits' can be hard to break so you will need to maintain the change in practice over a reasonable time period. The final aspect of the process is to collect evidence that allows you to evaluate the impact that the changes have made in practice.

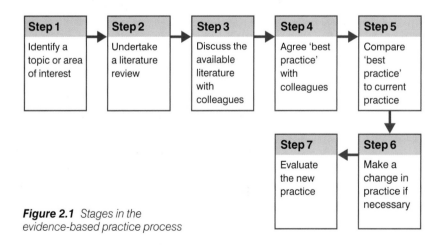

Figure 2.1 *Stages in the evidence-based practice process*

Understanding the stages of implementing evidence-based practice is not all that is required for effective evidence-based practice to occur. Health-care professionals also need leadership and support from their organisation, appraisal skills to identify the potential risks and benefits involved in implementing changes and the skills of critiquing research.

What is clinical audit?

Audit has a lot in common with research. It also involves systematically collecting information and, like evidence-based practice and health-care research, is about improving patient care. The key differences between research, evidence-based practice and audit are:

- **Research** leads to new knowledge, answering questions such as 'What should we do in our future practice?'

- **Evidence-based practice** is clinical practice based on the best knowledge available. It answers questions such as 'What practice is best supported through strong evidence?'

- **Audit** examines whether the best existing knowledge is really informing what actually occurs in practice. It answers questions such as 'How successful are we in what we do for the patient, compared to the standard we would like?'

Audit does not, therefore, tell us whether changes in the patient's health are directly due to the clinical interventions or practices examined. Auditing practice involves comparing what should be happening with what is really happening and, having identified a gap between the two, taking action to reduce the gap. Audit occurs in a cyclical way (Figure 2.2).

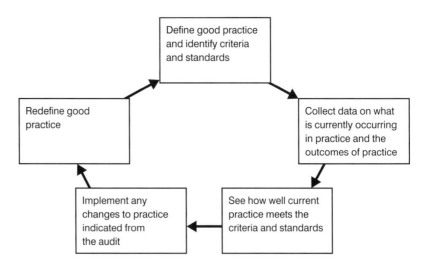

Figure 2.2 *The audit cycle*

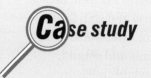

Case study

Ayesha's stoma care study

Ayesha is a stoma care nurse. She is a specialist nurse who works with patients having surgery that involves part of their intestine being removed. This sometimes leads to them having the intestine brought onto the surface of the abdomen and the contents being discharged into a disposable bag. She is going to undertake an audit regarding preparation of patients who are having a planned operation to form a stoma. She is setting up an audit and has written the standard below.

Stoma care standard

Topic	Stoma care nursing
Subtopic	Pre-operative preparation of planned admission patients who are to undergo stoma surgery
Standard	All patients who are to undergo stoma surgery (planned) should be given preoperative information that adequately prepares them for their impending operation by a stoma nurse or a registered nurse with the relevant knowledge

Structure

A stoma nurse will be available to see patients who are to undergo planned stoma care surgery

Registered nurses will be available on all general surgical wards who have adequate stoma care knowledge and have spent time working with the stoma care team

Stoma care literature for staff and patients should be available on all general surgical wards

A selection of stoma appliances should be available to show patients

Names and contact addresses of people with stomas willing to meet with patients should be available to staff who are preparing patients preoperatively

Process

1 The stoma nurse (registered nurse with relevant knowledge) should meet with the patient prior to surgery and outline their role

2 Provide opportunity to discuss patient problems and worries, allowing sufficient time and privacy

3 The surgery should be explained in a clear and carefully worded way, and diagrams and illustrations should be referred to

4 The patient should be given stoma care literature, which they can read on their own

5 If the patient is comfortable with this, the family or significant others should be invited and included in information-giving sessions

6 If the patient is comfortable with this, a suitable visitor who has had a similar operation should be introduced

7 Suitable appliances should be shown to the patient, and one fitted and appropriately sited

8 The stoma should be sited where it can be seen and reached by the patient, as well as positioned to allow adequate adhesion for the appliance

9 The need for bowel preparation and dietary management preoperatively should be explained

Outcome

That all patients who are to undergo planned stoma surgery are offered and given sufficient pre-operative information

That all patients who are to undergo planned stoma surgery perceive that they were adequately prepared for their surgery

At the beginning of the audit cycle the clinical team needs to decide what to measure. To do this, they identify the criteria and standards that are seen to be important in delivering quality of care. Usually, this will be decided by a group of professionals and clients and should, where possible, be based on research findings. Standards measure a desired level of achievement, almost like a baseline for practice. The criteria are a set of statements that break down achievement of the standard into measurable parts.

Typically, clinical auditors focus on:

- **Structure**: facilities, organisation, resources
- **Process**: behaviour, carrying out the treatment or care
- **Outcome**: patients' behaviour, knowledge, health status, satisfaction.

Data is then collected to find out how often (and how well) these criteria and standards are achieved in practice. If the audit data identifies situations where standards are not met, appropriate changes to the service are made to redefine and re-establish standards, and the cycle can begin again.

Reflective activity

Developing and evaluating a standard

- Can you see a way that the criteria in Ayesha's standard could be written to make them easier to measure?
- What methods do you think Ayesha could use to audit evidence on the application of the various criteria in the standard with the patients she cares for?

What ideas did you come up with? Perhaps you thought that a minimum amount of time to be spent giving the patient information should be included in the criteria. You might also have thought about stating the particular patient leaflets that should be given. In terms of evaluation, you might have suggested giving patients a questionnaire a few days after surgery, or using a checklist to be kept with the patient's care records that identifies when, what, how and by whom information was given to individual patients.

You can see how some of the same data collection tools used in research might be used in a clinical audit. You will also now understand why clinical audit is not research.

*RRRRR***Rapid recap**

Check your progress so far by working through each of the following questions.

1. How does evidence-based practice differ from simply using the findings of a research study in practice?
2. Why is it sometimes difficult to get research findings used to improve practice?
3. What does the term 'clinical audit' mean?

If you have difficulty with more than one of the questions, read through the section again to refresh your understanding before moving on.

References

NHS Executive (1996) *Promoting clinical effectiveness; A framework for action in and through the NHS*. Department of Health, London.

Sackett, D., Rosenburg, W., Gray, J. *et al.* (1996) Evidence-based medicine: what it is and what it isn't. *British Medical Journal,* **312**, 71–72.

Further reading

Bury, T. and Mead, J. (1998) *Evidence-based Healthcare: A practical guide for therapists*. Butterworth-Heinemann, Oxford.

Le May, A. (1999) *Evidence-based Practice*. Nursing Times Monograph 1. Emap Healthcare, London.

Renfrew, M. (1997) The development of evidence-based practice. *British Journal of Midwifery,* **5**, 100–104.

Types of
research investigation

When you read or hear people talk about research, you will come across a number of terms to identify different types of research investigation. The diagram below (Figure 3.1) groups types of research under four different headings for simplicity of explanation.

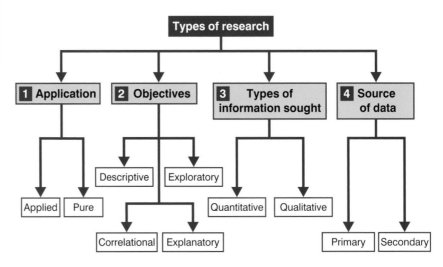

Figure 3.1 *Types of research*

Application

One way of understanding research is to consider what the methods are being applied to – abstract, theoretical ideas or practical issues.

Pure research

Pure (or basic) research tends to be conceptual rather than practical. It focuses on developing and testing theories and abstract ideas. Pure research may not have any practical application when it is conducted. This type of research is done to enlarge knowledge and understanding for its own sake. This does not mean that it is any less worthwhile than applied research. It may, in fact, result in theoretical developments that enable other applied research to be carried out at some time in the future, and it can also help to develop an understanding of phenomena, issues or problems at a theoretical level.

Applied research

Applied research is common in the health and social sciences, and is arguably a more appropriate focus for a student research project than pure research. This type of research applies theories and research methods to real situations, problems or issues. The findings of applied research are usually used for a practical purpose, such as making recommendations for new policies, improving practices or procedures or extending understanding of a particular situation.

Objectives

A second way of understanding research is to consider what it seeks to do. Kumar (1996) suggests that research can broadly do one or more of four different things. It can try to:

- Describe something (for example, a situation, problem or practice): this is obviously *descriptive research* – the researcher tries to describe (paint a mental picture of) the findings derived from careful, systematic collection and recording of data
- Establish the links or relationships between two factors (usually called *variables*): this is called *correlational research*
- Explain how and why a link or relationship exists between two factors (those variables again!): this is called *explanatory research* and tends to be seeking an answer to a specific question identified at the start of the research
- Investigate a poorly understood topic: this type of research study is called *exploratory research* – research questions in this type of study are often broad-ranging and the precise research focus develops throughout the research.

Health-care student research projects often involve a combination of the above types of research. For example, you could begin a study with an exploratory component to assess or refine your data collection procedures. You might then collect descriptive data on your chosen subject. This might lead you to extend your study by testing a theory about links between variables in the situation.

Exploratory pilot research might be conducted into the nursing handover of information from one shift of nurses to the new shift

Keywords

Quantitative
Quantitative research is usually concerned with the collection and analysis of data that focus on numbers, frequencies and trends

when they come on duty. General observations about what happens during handover ('What do nurses actually do?') could provide the basis for further study. The exploratory study would provide some ideas about what could be researched and what might be interesting.

Descriptive research might be conducted to extend knowledge about the different forms of handover. Descriptive researchers simply outline (describe) what they observe, answering the question 'What is happening here?' This type of research can often be the starting-point for further studies that ask 'Why' questions.

Correlational research might involve a study that investigates whether nurses use handover times to team-build. Correlational research simply establishes whether a link between the two variables – time spent on handover and teamworking – actually exists. A correlational study could explain *whether* there is a relationship between these two variables, but it wouldn't explain *why* or *how* this develops or works.

Explanatory research might involve a study that examines the why and how questions about the communications developed within handover. Research questions might include 'How do nurses use humour to reduce stress levels within handover?' or 'Why are long verbal handovers used to communicate between shifts?' This kind of research is often looking for causes.

The type of information sought

A third way of describing research is to consider the type of data being sought.

Quantitative

A **quantitative** study seeks numerical data. Some researchers set out to collect data that measures how many, how often, what percentage or proportion or 'To what extent is there a connection between x and y?' When the data has been collected, statistical techniques are used to establish and describe the numerical patterns and relationships that exist in the data. Quantitative research always involves measuring in some way.

Qualitative

Not all data are reducible to a numerical form and researchers do not always want to collect measurements of things. For example, a lot of health-care research is conducted into people's experiences.

O—π *Keywords*

Qualitative
Qualitative research is mainly
descriptive and involves
the collection and analysis
of data about meanings,
attitudes and beliefs

This produces non-numerical **qualitative** data. Those who use
a naturalistic approach to investigate people's feelings and beliefs,
or ways of life, find qualitative data in a variety of sources and
are interested in appreciating the meanings attached to them.
Research investigations that are primarily seeking these
non-numerical forms of data are often called *qualitative studies*.

The source of the data

A fourth – and our final – way of classifying a research investigation is to
identify the main source of the data. The term 'data' simply refers to the
items of information that are produced through research. For example,
when using a questionnaire, the data that a researcher collects are
the answers that each respondent gives to the questions asked.

Primary sources

Imagine that you were asked to carry out research into the bonding
and relationship development between a mother and her new-born
baby. Where could you get data on this? One strategy would be to
get permission to go with midwives into homes and midwifery units
and observe what happens. The data that you would actually collect
yourself by doing this is known as *primary data*. This kind of data
is new, original research information that is directly obtained by
the researcher.

Secondary sources

An alternative kind of research information is *secondary data*.
It may be more appropriate for your research study into mothers'
bonding with their new babies to look at sources of data that already
exist on this topic. The midwives may have made notes in their records
about mother and baby bonding and the relationships that develop.
The department may already have developed policies about the
environment to increase and improve mother–baby interaction. It is
also possible that somebody else, perhaps a professional researcher,
has already carried out a similar study and produced some useful data.
You might also find some statistics on breast-feeding as an aspect
of mother and baby bonding that you could use in your study.
All these pre-existing sources provide what is known as *secondary
data*. Researchers do not produce the data personally but obtain it
as a second-hand report or record and then reuse it in their own
research study.

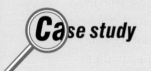

Case study

Davina's health promotion project

For her health promotion project Davina studied what young men knew and thought about alcohol consumption (binge drinking and social drinking). She used a variety of sources of secondary data in her study. Davina began by looking through newspapers for recent stories about men and alcohol consumption, and obtained some statistics on young men involved in road accidents related to drink-driving. She also used some psychology and biology books to find out about and make notes on the effects of alcohol on physical co-ordination and thinking.

Davina then carried out three interviews about drinking and driving with male students on her course. She used information from these interviews to identify key sub-topics and issues relating to drink driving. Davina then explored the subtopics and issues with a sample of male students at her higher education institute not on a health-care course, using a questionnaire.

First-time researchers often make a lot of use of secondary data, using it to provide a significant amount of evidence on their research topic and supporting it with a limited amount of their own primary data. Experienced researchers, however, tend to put a greater focus on primary research, supporting their own data with a more limited amount of relevant secondary research. You should not, however, see secondary research as less important than primary research. What is actually important is making an appropriate choice of data collection method for the topic you choose to investigate.

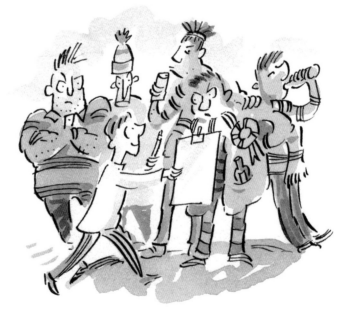

Choosing the right moment to collect primary data is an important research skill

There are a variety of ways in which you could use secondary data sources in a research investigation. For example, you might use secondary sources to find out what has already been researched on the topic that is to be investigated. This would give some background information (literature review). When writing up a research report the findings can be compared with existing (secondary) data on the same topic.

RRRRRRapid recap

Check your progress so far by working through each of the following questions.

1. What is the difference between pure and applied research?
2. What does descriptive research set out to do?
3. What are researchers who conduct correlation research looking for?
4. What kind of research asks 'How' and 'Why' questions?
5. Can you give two examples of secondary data sources that a researcher might use?
6. How does primary data differ from secondary data?
7. What term would be used to describe numerical information obtained by a researcher?

If you have difficulty with more than one of the questions, read through the section again to refresh your understanding before moving on.

References

Kumar, R. (1996) *Research Methodology*. Sage Publications, London.

Further reading

Carr L. (1994) The strengths and weaknesses of quantitative and qualitative research: what method for nursing? *Journal of Advanced Nursing,* **20**, 716–721.

Duffy, M. (1985) Designing nursing research: the qualitative–quantitative debate. *Journal of Advanced Nursing,* **10**, 225–232.

4

The role of theory in research

Learning outcomes

By the end of this chapter you should be able to:

- Discuss the main differences between positivist and naturalistic approaches to research

- Appreciate the role of theory in research

- Understand why a particular theoretical approach is used in a research study

Theoretical approaches to research

If you had to do a small-scale research study, the idea of taking a theoretical approach to your research investigation might seem a little bit daunting at first. It is useful, however, for you to understand that any research investigation requires the researcher to adopt a particular theoretical perspective or viewpoint. Do not worry about the academic terms – 'adopting a theoretical perspective' is not as difficult as it sounds. Basically, there are two choices. Researchers can adopt either a *positivist* approach or a *naturalistic* approach.

The theoretical approach chosen enables researchers to make links between their own beliefs about what constitutes useful and valid 'knowledge' ('How is it possible to understand the world?') and the practical issue of actually obtaining research data.

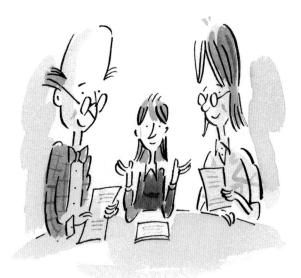

You won't need an extra large brain to use theory in your research. A little bit of careful thinking is usually enough

An understanding of the theoretical approach should drive the data collection methods and general design of the research. If the theoretical approach is not considered adequately, this can lead to inconsistencies and shortcomings in the research.

The positivist approach

The positivist approach to research investigation is commonly used in the natural sciences (physics, chemistry and biology). It is also widely used by psychology, medical and health-care researchers and is sometimes referred to as the *scientific approach*.

Positivist theory is based on a number of key assumptions. It is claimed that:

- Researchers can discover and measure true 'facts' about the world
- Methods used to study the physical world can be modified and used to study the social world
- Only 'knowledge' gained through observed experience is valid and 'scientific'
- Research that is carried out in a controlled and rigorous way enables scientific 'truths' to be discovered
- The researcher can, and should, avoid having any personal influence on the research process.

Researchers who accept the basic assumptions of positivism tend to choose data collection methods such as questionnaires, structured interviews and observational checklists, because these allow them to collect 'facts' in a controlled way. These 'facts' tend to be recorded in, or are reducible to, a numerical form. Numerical items of information are often referred to as *quantitative data*.

Positivist researchers typically try to test and observe relationships between *variables*. Natural or physical variables are the characteristics of entities that can be physically manipulated, such as the heat or volume of a substance. For example, the volume of alcohol that a person is able to consume before becoming unconscious is a variable that is related, in part, to the person's body mass. Larger, heavier people can generally consume more alcohol than smaller, lighter people because of their greater body mass. *Social variables* are attributes that are assigned to people and that occur in different levels, strengths or amounts within the population. For example, marital status is a social variable that varies in terms of whether a person is single, married or divorced.

Researchers who adopt a positivist approach usually try to control the variables that they study. They do this so that they can identify 'cause and effect' relationships between variables. The classic 'controlled' research strategy is the laboratory experiment. Medical researchers, for example, frequently use controlled laboratory experiments to develop and test the effects of new medicines. They use this approach to identify the positive and negative effects that their new medicines cause in the controlled experimental situation.

Researchers who collect data by conducting laboratory experiments impose a high level of control over the research situation, so that they are able to say with certainty how the relationship between the variables works. They are looking for scientific 'truths'. Scientific truths are things that always happen or that apply under specific conditions. A belief in the assumptions of positivism allows researchers to claim that their findings can be *generalised*. In other words, they believe that their findings are 'true facts' that can be applied from the research setting to the world in general.

People who put together questionnaires, interviews with pre-arranged questions or observation checklists with predefined observation categories are also trying to control the research situation that they are studying. They are also setting limits and boundaries on the possible sources and nature of the data that is collected, by deciding in advance what they will ask about, look for or test.

Within health care an experimental, positivistic approach may not be appropriate or possible. In these instances a researcher may choose what is termed a *quasi-experimental* approach. Quasi-experimental studies involve examining the relationship between something that is being altered or changed (e.g. a new activities programme in a care-of-the-older-person setting) and the eventual outcome of this (length of social interactions between elderly patients/clients). However, unlike true positivistic, experimental designs, certain aspects of control are absent, such as the possibility of allocating patients to a control group who do not receive the new activities programme. Instead, observational measurements might be made prior to the introduction of the new programme, immediately following its introduction and 3 months later. This method of gathering data is sometimes called a *pre-test/post-test* design.

Researchers who adopt a positivist approach put great store in maintaining a distance between themselves as 'research experts' and what happens in the research setting or situation itself. They adopt the position of very interested, but outside, observers of the events

☍🗝 Keywords

Grounded theory
An inductive approach to qualitative data that requires the findings to be firmly 'grounded' in the data, so prior theoretical findings are avoided as far as possible. In using this method, the researcher will not undertake a full literature review prior to undertaking the data collection. Data collection is undertaken in parallel with analysis. Categories or themes identified are provisional and may be modified.
(Glaser and Strauss 1987)

that they are studying. Researchers who adopt a positivist approach feel that this is necessary in order to protect their objectivity and avoid influencing, or being influenced by, the people or events that they are studying.

The naturalistic approach

The naturalistic approach to research investigation developed out of criticism of some of the claims and weaknesses of the positivist approach. The naturalistic approach is strongly associated with the disciplines of anthropology and sociology. In health-care-related research it is likely to be used by members of non-medical disciplines, such as social workers, nurses and occupational therapists, who want to understand the experiences of the individuals and groups that they study.

Naturalistic researchers tend to look in detail at a specific group of people or a particular situation. They do not try to discover scientific 'truths' or establish causal relationships. The naturalistic approach is based on the idea that 'knowledge' is something that people create continuously, and that no fixed, objective reality exists independently of people's culture, values and experience. *Social constructivists* believe that reality is assembled as people interact within a particular context. There are, therefore, multiple realities rather than one single objective reality. As a result, researchers using naturalistic approaches do not set out to collect generalisable 'facts'. They try to gain an awareness and appreciation of how particular individuals or groups of people view and experience the world.

Researchers adopting a naturalistic approach base their data collection strategy on the assumption that their main task is to understand reality from the 'inside', from the perspective of the 'researched'. Naturalistic researchers are interested in the real meaning of human behaviour and relationships, and believe that this can only be discovered and understood in the natural setting where it occurs. As a result, naturalistic researchers tend to use data collection methods such as 'participant observation' and unstructured in-depth interviews, which allow them to gain access to a wide variety of non-numerical qualitative data. A researcher adopting a naturalistic approach might be interested in what people say and communicate, what they do in different situations and how they look and present themselves. All these data are non-numerical but, if researchers can appreciate the meaning and significance of the information, it may help them to understand what's going on.

Theory and **Practice**

The choice of qualitative or quantitative approach depends on the research question. Some researchers use both qualitative and quantitative approaches. One method is not better than another.

Two examples of naturalistic perspectives to undertaking research are ethnography and phenomenology.

Ethnography involves the researcher participating in the lives of those being researched, collecting data in order to provide an explanation for the research topic chosen. The researcher seeks to understand the culture of the people being studied and observes this in the natural setting. The naturalistic findings from this type of research are basically descriptive. *Phenomenology*, on the other hand, is more interpretive and tries to understand the social issue or human activity being studied from the viewpoint of people's perceptions of their own experiences.

Most researchers who adopt a naturalistic approach accept that they inevitably play a part in the research situation, and that they should acknowledge this in the way in which they set up, conduct and write up their research investigations. This does not mean that the naturalistic approach allows a researcher to deliberately manipulate the participants or bias their findings. It means that they must find ways of identifying and acknowledging how factors such as their existing social characteristics, experiences and culture may affect what it is possible for them to see, understand and experience in the research setting. For example, the existing beliefs and values of the researcher are seen to play an important role in influencing their decisions about what are 'important', 'interesting' and 'useful' data.

Deciding which approach to adopt

While it is possible to distinguish and criticise both the positivist and naturalistic approaches to research, you should beware of 'joining a side', as it were, and becoming a positivist or a naturalistic researcher forever! In practice, researchers can use both approaches, either at different stages in a research investigation (see 'Triangulation – covering all bases' in Chapter 10, p.104) or over a series of studies. Both positivist and naturalistic approaches are useful and necessary for research in the health, social and psychological sciences. Researchers always make judgements about which is the most appropriate approach to use, taking into account the circumstances that they are working in, their subject matter and what they are trying to achieve. One of the first tasks in planning a research investigation is to determine the theoretical approach that underpins the study.

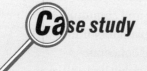

Case study

Simon's dissertation

Simon works as an occupational therapist linked to a care-of-the-older-person rehabilitation ward. For his dissertation he wants to undertake a research project about promoting independence for patients. He's interested in the possible impact that encouraging older people to do their own washing and dressing has on their sense of independence.

Simon has found some previous research on this topic by doing a literature review. It indicates that rehabilitation interventions with patients can be time-consuming and that certain communication strategies have a positive part to play in rehabilitation.

From a positivist theoretical perspective he could research the impact of the number of staff in the ward involved in care delivery in a morning shift and the time spent in washing and dressing patients. He could observe, measure and compare the nurse and occupational therapist activities with patients, using an observational checklist identifying the time spent promoting independence in these daily activities. From a naturalistic approach he could undertake in-depth interviews with staff, investigating their attitudes and feelings about patient independence and their views on how they think it is best to promote this. Alternatively, he could record participant observational data regarding the promotion of independence in washing and dressing.

Simon's choice regarding his approach to the research will partly be determined by how focused his topic becomes, by his own beliefs and values regarding positivistic and naturalistic approaches to research and by his abilities and opportunity to use certain data collection methods.

Reflective activity

If you were in Simon's situation what theoretical approach (positivistic or naturalistic) would you take?
What sources of data would you use? (primary or secondary or both)
Reflect carefully on your reasons for making these choices.

What is the role of theory in research?

Positivistic and naturalistic approaches are forms of theory that influence research studies. It is useful to examine here the place of theory in research study.

Theory is a central element in all the forms of research already examined. Research can build on existing theories, exploring and developing them (*theory testing*) or can identify new theories (*theory building*). The processes we use to understand and make sense of 'reality' are shaped by concepts that provide tags or labels for the 'things' (for example, objects, events, experiences – 'desk', 'blood pressure' or 'mental illness') that constitute our world. Concepts allow us to organise our understanding and communicate this to each other. Theory therefore acts as an explanatory framework that provides understanding about a related set of concepts.

Leon Festinger, a psychologist, developed and published a theory that he called 'cognitive dissonance theory' in 1957. This theory states that, where there is a mismatch between your beliefs and your own behaviour, you will experience a feeling of discomfort. The theory also goes on to state that people tend to change their beliefs rather than their behaviour in an attempt to resolve this tension. Although this may be the case, 'cognitive dissonance theory' is rather generalised and abstract.

In order to develop his theory, Festinger decided to test it. He undertook a whole range of research investigations to explore situations where a person's beliefs ran counter to their actions. For example, suppose an individual has a belief that, when they spend a large sum of money, they should make sure this is a well-thought-through decision. Festinger found that, following a decision to buy an expensive object, such as a car, on purely personal liking or through impulse decision-making, the buyer would indulge in activities to reduce 'cognitive dissonance'. They might seek literature about levels of fuel consumption and comparisons to other cars and might take more notice of information that supported their original acquisition. In this way, any discomfort or 'cognitive dissonance' caused by spending a large sum of money without fully examining the options can be reduced.

A health-care researcher might use the framework of 'cognitive dissonance' theory to support a study on nurse managers' behaviour. They might discover that 'cognitive dissonance' occurred because of a conflict between the nurse manager's belief that registered nurses should deliver nursing care and a skill mix problem that meant that, because of a limited staffing budget, much of the nursing care was delivered by health-care support workers. How can nurse managers resolve the 'cognitive dissonance' that occurs? One solution is that nurse managers might seek opportunities to change their beliefs. For example they might begin paying more attention to thank you letters from patients that identify the good care provided by health-care support workers, and might become more actively involved in training them.

Through the previous discussion you can see how theory plays an important part in research and can also be the outcome of research.

Hopefully you will now feel a bit more comfortable with using the terms 'concept' and 'theory'. As you read more research and undertake your own you will understand more about the role that theory plays in your health-care practice.

Over to you

Find a piece of research from a journal. Read it and try to identify where the researcher has used theory.

Did the research have a theoretical framework?

Was the research positivistic or naturalistic?

Does the research build theory or test theory?

RRRRRRapid recap

Check your progress so far by working through each of the following questions.

1. If a researcher is gathering data using a structured questionnaire that allows numerical analysis, what is the likely theoretical approach adopted for the research?
2. A researcher is collecting data through observing biology lecturers teaching on health-care courses as they go about their everyday work. What is the likely theoretical approach underpinning this research?
3. Identify the difference between the terms theory testing and theory building.

If you have difficulty with more than one of the questions, read through the section again to refresh your understanding before moving on.

References

Festinger, L. (1957) *A Theory of Cognitive Dissonance*. Tavistock, London.

Glaser, B and Strauss, A (1967) *The Discovery of Grounded Theory: Strategies for qualitative research*. Aldine Press, Chicago.

Further reading

Creswell, J. (1998) *Qualitative Inquiry and Research Design: Choosing among five traditions*. Sage, Thousand Oaks, CA.

Sim, J. and Wright, C. (2000) *Research in Health Care: Concepts, designs and methods*. Stanley Thornes, Cheltenham, pp. 5–14.

5

Reading and judging research

Learning outcomes

By the end of this chapter you should be able to:

- Discuss the criteria used to judge research studies
- Discriminate between the terms 'validity' and 'reliability'
- Outline how in evidence-based practice the strength of the evidence is affected by the research design
- Explain how systematic reviews and clinical guidelines are used in practice

A research report is evaluated in terms of the following criteria:

- The reliability of the data collection methods used
- The validity of the data collected
- The representativeness of the research sample or setting used
- The objectivity of the researcher
- The ethical standards of the research.

All these issues need to be considered at some time during the planning and carrying out of a research study. When reading research you need to judge whether the researcher has demonstrated a considered response to the issues identified above. In this chapter we will look at each of these criteria, except ethics. The ethical aspects of research are covered in Chapter 11 as a separate topic .

Reliability

When we say that something 'is reliable' or 'can be relied on' we tend to mean that it consistently works in a very general sense. The term *reliability* has a more precise meaning within research and is about reproducing consistent data. Patrick McNeill (1990) says that 'if a method of collecting evidence is reliable, it means that anybody else using this method, or the same person using it at another time, would come up with the same findings'. When you are reading research or developing a research project you need to feel confident that the data collection methods are reliable. To judge reliability when reading a research study you need to determine not only whether the method was reliable but also whether this was the best method to gather data for the subject being studied. Some data collection methods are seen to be more reliable than others. Data collection methods that involve researchers working on their own, in situations that cannot be replicated (repeated), and where researchers use their beliefs, values or preconceptions to decide which 'data' are important, tend to be less reliable than data collection methods that do not have these characteristics.

There are three main aspects of reliability.

- The **equivalence** of a research tool (such as a questionnaire) is concerned with whether it produces consistent measurements when used by two different researchers or by the same researcher in two different settings. Equivalence might be a factor if you had a 'quality of life following breast surgery questionnaire', which you might want to adapt to use in a 'quality of life following hip replacement surgery' study.

- **Stability or repeatability** is concerned with how consistently the research tool measures the same thing when it is used on repeated occasions.

- **Internal consistency** is a term for determining whether the individual parts of a tool are also reliable. For instance, a questionnaire might include three questions that are meant to measure attitudes towards people who deliberately harm themselves. If all three questions receive high, or low, scores for being accepting of people who self-harm, then internal consistency is likely to be good. If the completed questionnaires show that the first two questions receive a high score and the third a low score, the third question may not be measuring attitudes to people who self-harm but something else.

Validity

Using unreliable data collection methods or tools leads to validity problems with the data.

This concept refers to the issue of whether the data collected is a 'true' picture of what is being studied. There are many reasons why the data that a researcher collects can be 'invalid'. For example, the data can be a product of the research instrument used rather than a true 'picture', or indicator, of what they are actually claimed to be. It is relatively straightforward and easy to show that thermometers only measure temperature (hot/cold), but we can be much less certain of the validity of a tool to measure social variables such as 'quality of life' or intelligence (such as IQ – intelligence quotient – tests). Do they really measure what they claim to measure?

The issue regarding IQ tests is all about their ability and effectiveness to give a true, independent measurement of intelligence. Intelligence tests have been shown to be quite reliable in that, if the same IQ test is used on repeated occasions with the same person, it is very likely to produce the same findings each time. This does not mean that such tests give *valid* findings, just that they are *reliable* at measuring whatever it is that they are actually measuring. The validity of IQ tests is questioned on the grounds that they really only reveal how good a person is at doing IQ tests – and not the true level of the person's IQ.

Similarly, the validity of the data acquired through using questionnaires and interviews could be challenged on the grounds that respondents may give answers that are not actually true. Such data may lack validity if the respondents deliberately lie, or give answers that do not actually represent how they behave in reality. For example, people who complete questionnaires or take part in research interviews will usually say that they are non-sexist and non-racist, and may well believe that this is true. While they may not be deliberately lying, their real behaviour – at work and with their friends, for example – may reveal something about their beliefs that they do not wish to acknowledge or admit. For both the above reasons, the validity of questionnaire and interview data should never be taken for granted or relied upon.

The reliability of data collection methods and the validity of the data obtained are always important issues to consider when evaluating your own research or the conclusions that others arrive at when they publish research findings. A third factor that must be taken into account when judging the quality of a research investigation is the representativeness of the data sources.

Representativeness

McNeill (1990) says that representativeness 'refers to the question of whether the group or situation being studied are typical of others'. If a group or situation is representative of others, then researchers can *generalise* their findings. That is, they can say that what's true for this group or situation is true of others. If we do not know whether the group or situation is representative, it is not safe, or correct, to claim that the research findings can be generalised beyond the group or situation that has been studied. Researchers who want to generalise their findings use various sampling methods (see Chapter 9) to try to ensure that their research is based on a representative group of people or a representative situation.

There are also many situations in which researchers do not use sampling methods and acknowledge that their findings cannot be generalised. For example, researchers who use participant observation

Keywords

Transparency
The belief that researchers' interpretations of experimental evidence should be available to be checked, examined, critiqued and used as a basis for convincing others that the research findings are valid

(see Chapter 10) or case study (see Chapter 9) methods do not usually seek to study a representative group or situation and so do not use sampling techniques.

Representativeness is much more important an issue if a positivist rather than a naturalistic approach to the research investigation is adopted. This does not mean that if a naturalistic approach is taken the issue can be ignored. People reading research reports still need to consider whether the data sources are representative, and they should expect to see how the responses taken by the researcher relate to the problems that other naturalistic researchers face in this area. At the very least, a justification should be given for not seeking or using a representative sample of people or research setting in an investigation (see Chapter 13).

Objectivity

Researchers should be objective, as opposed to biased or prejudiced, in the way that they carry out their investigations. Researchers must suspend their pre-existing judgements and view the research situation and the research problem from the viewpoint of 'a stranger'. Researchers who are trying to be objective avoid letting their values, beliefs and pre-existing ideas affect or influence the way in which they develop a project, conduct research or analyse the data.

Some researchers, particularly if they adopt a naturalistic approach, feel that it is impossible to be truly objective when conducting research. They argue that researchers inevitably introduce aspects of their 'self' into the research process. The answer to this, for naturalistic researchers, is to acknowledge their role in, and possible influence on, the research process when they are writing up their account of the research investigation. When researchers reflect on their own assumptions and actions through the research process, this is termed the process of *reflexivity*.

In order to be objective, researchers must be open and 'public' in the way that they conduct and explain their research. In the final research report and presentation, it is important to show clearly how the research was conducted, to present the data in an accessible way and to justify any conclusions that have been reached. This allows other interested parties to check whether the research has been acceptably conducted and evaluate whether the conclusions that have been drawn are valid and reliable. Objectivity and openness reduce the risk of reaching false conclusions, deliberately or accidentally, by conducting a flawed piece of research. In part, objectivity relates to the ethical issue of the researcher being honest. This and other 'ethical' aspects of research investigations are discussed further in the section on research ethics.

How do you judge between different research articles?

There is often a great deal of research and evidence on a particular aspect of patient care or treatment. In this book you have already been introduced to the term evidence-based practice. To support your health-care practice by evidence you will need to be able to compare different forms of evidence. Once you have obtained a range of research evidence the next step is to 'grade' or determine the strength of the research. The strength of evidence on which to base a clinical decision varies from topic to topic. In evidence-based practice the evidence gathered by certain research methods are perceived to be stronger. The stronger evidence is able to meet the criteria already discussed in terms of reliability, validity, representativeness and objectivity. The types of evidence and their relative strengths are listed below with (1) being the strongest and (4) the weakest.

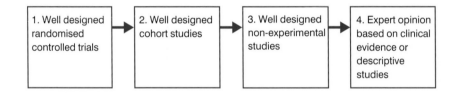

Figure 5.1 *The hierarchy of strength of evidence*

The highest level or strongest evidence (1) is obtained from a *randomised controlled trial* (RCT) and this is often used in medicine. It involves an experimental design comparing the outcomes between two or more groups randomly assigned to a treatment/intervention group versus another strategy/no treatment group. To reduce the possibility of distortion of the results of the research, the researchers and all patients participate 'blind'. This means that they do not know which group is receiving the treatment/intervention being examined. Within the hierarchy of evidence, RCTs are considered to be the 'gold standard' for evidence-based medicine as they are able to produce the strongest research evidence.

The next level of evidence includes experiments without randomisation, for example, a study of one cohort or group of patients who have been given the treatment.

Non-experimental research is placed lower in the hierarchy of research evidence, with expert opinions being viewed as the lowest level of evidence upon which to base clinical decisions.

Nursing and other health-care professions have developed a varied research tradition using a wide variety of research methods and designs. RCTs, for instance, are infrequently used as a research design in nursing studies. Using the hierarchy above would prove challenging in many instances when you review the evidence to support your practice, as evidence-based practice relies on the different types of evidence that professionals have available.

How do systematic reviews of research and clinical guidelines help research to be used in practice?

Even if research is available, this may not lead to the findings being used in practice settings. Busy health-care practitioners may not have the time to carefully judge a wide range of research findings, so they may just carry on giving care or treatment in the same way. In the UK there has been a trend towards the increased production of rigorously created, research-based information in the form of systematic reviews and clinical guidelines. This means that the judging of which research evidence to use has already been done for the health-care practitioner.

Systematic reviews summarise all the available research evidence on a given area using a rigorous approach across a number of research studies. This ensures that variations between studies and contradictory results can be understood within a single conclusion. Systematic reviews are often conducted by a group of experts. If you are able to find a systematic review on the area of practice you are investigating, this is really useful.

Clinical guidelines are written records, systematically developed and designed on the best evidence available at the time, which offer a guidance or recommendations for practice in a given situation. The process that transforms the evidence from a systematic review into a clinical guideline is termed *translation*. The aim of translation is to provide useful, usable and relevant ways of using evidence in a practice setting and in a way that suits your area of health-care work. It involves combining research evidence with ethical, organisational and other expert advice. There are quite a few different types of clinical guidelines and these broadly sit within three different groups.

Table 5.1 **Types of clinical guidelines**

Type	Definition
Algorithms, decision trees, flow charts	These consist of a formula or set of rules for dealing with a particular problem that prompts a decision
Care maps, clinical or critical pathways	These provide a guide for the care of patients with a particular diagnosis. Variations are reported and they can be individualised for a patient
Protocols	These are precise and detailed plans for a particular treatment or therapy. They are more detailed and defined than those above, and are agreed at a local, national or international level

Reflective activity

Clinical guidelines

Identify one example of a clinical guideline you have seen in use.

Which of the three types of clinical guideline definitions best suits what you have identified?

Where can you find systematic reviews and clinical guidelines?

Both systematic review and clinical guidelines form part of the research-based information and expert knowledge that is provided in an easily accessible format. Bodies such as the Cochrane Collaboration and the NHS Centre for Reviews and Dissemination have been set up to commission or produce reviews of research evidence. These reviews of research evidence, which are widely available, are an attempt to reduce the variability of health care. For example, an elderly woman admitted to an accident and emergency department following a fracture of her hip could receive very different care in two hospitals in the same county.

Variations in practice occur for two main reasons:

- There is no agreed best practice and practitioners have, therefore, to choose what they believe to be the best approach
- Best practice has been agreed through examination of the best available evidence but not all practitioners are aware of it.

One of the significant problems associated with evidence-based practice is the lack of well-defined research on many important aspects of health-care practice. It is therefore important that all health-care professions develop research skills and knowledge and the ability to judge the evidence.

RRRRRRapid recap

Check your progress so far by working through each of the following questions.

1. Name two things that weaken the reliability of a data collection method.
2. What does the concept of validity refer to?
3. Why can you not assume that interview data is 100% valid?
4. Explain why some researchers try to ensure that they select a representative sample of people for their research studies.
5. What are you if you are not objective?
6. What is termed the 'gold standard' of evidence-based practice?
7. What is the difference between a systematic review and a clinical guideline?

If you have difficulty with more than one of the questions, read through the section again to refresh your understanding before moving on.

Reference

McNeill, P. (1990) *Research Methods*. Routledge, London.

Further reading

De Vet de Bie, R., van der Heijden, G., Verhagen, A. *et al* (1997) Systematic reviews on the basis of methodological criteria. *Physiotherapy*, **83**, 284–289.

Magarey, J. (2001) Elements of a systematic review. *International Journal of Nursing Practice*, **7**, 376–382.

6 Identifying an area for research and developing a research question

How is a research topic or area of interest identified?

The research topic for a lot of health-care research is often determined by a 'commissioning' body such as the Department of Health or a pharmaceutical company, that pays for the research to be done. However, there is also a large body of research carried out by health-care practitioners who are particularly interested in an aspect of their practice. Sometimes, health-care practitioners do small-scale research studies as part of their studies. Within this chapter we will look at the early phases of the research process from your viewpoint as a first-time researcher making decisions about doing a small-scale research project.

Starting at the beginning, your first challenge is to identify a topic to research and, within that, a question to address. This is a creative part of the research process. You will need to think of some general ideas or topic areas that you are interested in researching. The idea that you end up with will have to be *researchable*. This means that the idea can be tested because you are able to obtain evidence about it.

Research process ▶ ▶ ▶ ▶

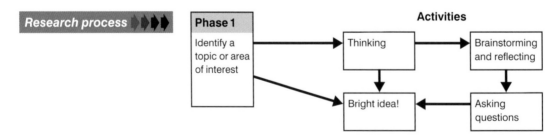

Figure 6.1 *Phase 1: Identifying a topic of interest*

Where do research ideas come from?

Basically, you need to have a bright idea. When researchers say that their bright idea 'just came to them', they are not telling you the whole story. Moments of creative insight and inspiration do result in breakthroughs for many people who are trying to think up a good research idea. However, these 'sudden' insights usually occur after the person has done a lot of thinking about different topics without making any apparent progress.

A good way of identifying possible topics to research is to spend some time talking to other students and staff on placements about the topics that you enjoy and that interest you. Then think about and sift through the ideas, experiences and interests that you have discussed. This will eventually lead to your moment of insight or breakthrough. You might come up with an idea because you have:

- Studied or learned about something that was exciting or interesting
- Read or heard about something that you believe is not true, or that you feel is an injustice
- Discovered a writer, topic or issue that particularly interests you
- Read about a research study that is intriguing, or that you question the validity of
- Always wanted to do a particular type of study, such as participant observation or in-depth interviews
- Have access to people who work in settings that are particularly interesting to you.

There is no magical or easy way to identify a research idea. Your bright idea is waiting to be identified – you have just got to find it! Remember that it is best to brainstorm and reflect on a range of possibilities before making your decision. Come up with several possibilities and then think them over.

Peter Langley (1993) suggests that you should ask the following questions about the ideas that you come up with:

- 'Is the proposed research **possible**?' That is, are you likely to be able to obtain primary and secondary data on the subject that you are interested in? Very specialist and sensitive topics may seem glamorous and exciting, but often it is not possible to obtain data on them. 'Management and behaviour of health-care staff in battle zones' might be interesting and potentially exciting, but you probably won't be able to get access to the data that you would need to make this project work.

- 'Is the idea **relevant** to your course?' The reason for your student research project is to develop and demonstrate your understanding of research skills as they relate to a particular subject area. Your project should, therefore, have strong links to the subject matter of your course. If it does not, your work may not be relevant to your course. Could you justify the 'battle zone' idea for your course?

- 'Is the project **interesting** enough to you?' You are probably going to be doing your research project for several months while still having to work in placement areas and at other studies. The topic that you choose should be interesting enough to motivate you to keep the project going until completion.

- 'Is the proposed research **ethically justifiable**?' That is, can you be sure that your research won't cause harm or offence, or get you into difficulties yourself? A project that involves any risk of harm to you or others cannot be justified (see Chapter 11 for further details on research ethics).

Reasons not to choose a topic

There are all sorts of reasons why you might be interested in a particular topic. One of the major problems that first-time researchers encounter is narrowing down the large number of topics that seem really interesting! However, you should definitely avoid some topics – including topics that are so personal to you that they provoke a very strong emotional reaction. You should consider avoiding issues where you have an 'axe to grind' or a very strong moral standpoint. Abortion and euthanasia are examples of topics that have big moral dimensions to them. The reason for avoiding them is that you may bring preconceived ideas and fairly fixed beliefs to the research. These are likely to limit your ability to work through the research process objectively.

The purpose of small-scale research is more about learning how to follow the research process effectively than about making scientific breakthroughs or startling discoveries about particular topics. You must avoid setting out on a project that is simply designed to confirm your preconceptions.

This does not mean that you should always avoid a topic simply because you have a standpoint, or have some kind of social, religious or political commitment relating to it. 'Standpoint research' is very common in the field of social policy, for example, and motivates many researchers who wish to make a difference to the aspects of society that they research. People who research poverty, mental distress and homelessness, for example, often declare their personal and professional commitment to helping people who are experiencing these problems. Feminist and antiracist researchers are also very committed 'standpoint' researchers, and focus on achieving particular social and political goals for women and minority ethnic groups who experience discrimination and disadvantage. However, while professional and academic researchers are expected to use their research experience and training to remain objective, first-time student researchers will find this much more difficult. You will need to strike a balance between committing yourself to a topic that interests and motivates you and being able to keep an open and objective mind about it.

'Decidophobia' and information overload

When you first try to come up with a research topic, you may experience some confusion and even feel overwhelmed by the task. Many first-time researchers do. It can feel a little like being lost. What you need is a sense of direction.

Finding an initial direction to go in is the key task of the early creative stages of your research project. Some people cannot think of any topics at first, while others think of too many possibilities and cannot decide between them – this is 'decidophobia'. The possibilities are infinite and this becomes a problem.

If you are finding it difficult to get started, or are becoming overwhelmed, a good 'way in' is to start off by thinking about the big topics that interest and motivate you in your course or area of work.

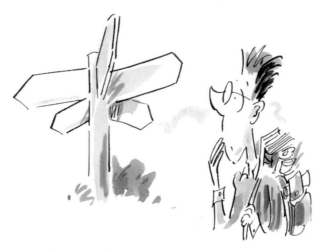

Choosing a 'big topic' will give your research direction

Reflective activity

Thinking big

You might like to fill in a copy of the 'Big ideas brainstorm' worksheet (Table 6.1) to complete this activity.

Brainstorm eight different big topics that you might be interested in exploring for your research study.

Think about your ideas for a while and decide which topics appeal most to you.

Reduce your brainstorm list by repeatedly discarding half of the ideas until you are left with the area that seems the most interesting one to you.

Table 6.1 **Big ideas brainstorm**

Possible topics	Second thoughts	Semi finalists	The winner!

Identify a general subject, or 'big topic' area that you are interested in, such as *health promotion, care of older people* or *mobility*, for example. Your 'big topic' will be a starting-point – the next step is to refine it.

It is impossible to identify a simple list of reasons why professional and academic researchers come up with their research ideas. Some researchers are driven by a personal desire or near obsession to investigate a new topic, or to investigate an established area in a way that nobody else has done before. Only they can explain why. As previously explained, however, in many other cases, researchers are commissioned, or asked, to conduct investigations by government and commercial organisations. In these circumstances, somebody else comes up with the idea or topic, and the researcher turns it into a research investigation.

Factors influencing the choice of your research topic:

- **Values**. Researchers' values can influence their choice of research topic and problem. Many sociologists and social policy academics have a strong belief in social justice and a commitment towards researching and exposing issues such as homelessness, poverty and unfair discrimination.

- **Knowledge gaps**. Many researchers choose their research topic because they believe that a gap exists in knowledge and understanding about it in their particular academic discipline or area of professional practice.

- **Solving problems and influencing policy**. Much health-care, psychological and social research focuses on solving problems, and is very practical in this sense. Believing that a social, psychological or health problem exists and ought to be dealt with is a significant motivation for some researchers in choosing their research topic.

- **Resources: time and money**. The amount of time and money that a researcher has available places some limitations on what s/he can do. As a first-time researcher you are unlikely to have either much time or much money to lavish on your research investigation. Simple matters such as printing and postage costs need to be taken into account at an early stage. Resource factors can ultimately influence fundamental decisions about the research strategy and methods that are used.

- **Enjoyment and interest**. These two factors should be high on your list of reasons for choosing a topic for your first research investigation. It is important that you choose a topic area that interests you, and that will contribute to the enjoyment that

Over to you

Identify possible research topics

Write down your responses to each prompt to demonstrate that you have thought through the various aspects involved in identifying a research topic.

Brainstorm a list of possible research topics.

Which were the most interesting?

Think about whether research on the topic is possible, relevant, meaningful and ethically justifiable.

Can you see any obvious problems in researching the topics that you have identified?

What factors have influenced your choice of research topic?

should be part of carrying out a research investigation. If you select a topic that is dull and uninteresting to you, you will find it hard to motivate yourself and complete the project when you hit a difficult patch, or are under pressure from this and other pieces of work that you have to do.

It seems that deciding on the research idea is solely down to you, but if you are doing research on your health-care course you will have an identified research supervisor, lecturer or tutor to go to. If you have other questions, doubts about or problems relating to choosing a research topic, you should talk them through with your tutor or supervisor at an early opportunity.

How do you identify a research question or hypothesis?

Phase 1 of your research project should have resulted in you identifying a 'big topic' to research. This is an important milestone in the life of your project – a breakthrough perhaps if you have struggled with 'decidophobia'. However, you will still need to do considerable work on your 'big topic' to turn it into a researchable one. This work is achieved in Phase 2 and involves carrying out a review of the background literature on your 'big topic' area. The aim of this is to allow you to focus more clearly on a specific aspect of the topic so that you can produce a clearly defined research question or hypothesis that will form the basis of the project. Phase 2 is covered in detail in Chapter 7 (page 49). You should also note at this point that many researchers continue to search literature sources after they have identified a research question or hypothesis. This allows them to continually update themselves to specific studies and theories that are relevant to their project. This should give you some sense of how the various phases of the research process tend to overlap each other rather than occurring in a clear cut step-by-step fashion.

So, how do you identify a research question or hypothesis when you have done an initial review of the background literature? You have two things to do. First you need to focus on a specific aspect of the topic that you have chosen. Then you need to focus on a 'problem' within it so that you can ask a clear question about it or state a hypothesis that can be investigated.

The research question that you choose shouldn't be too wide or too narrow. 'How many physiotherapy students training in England are studying physiotherapy in the county where they went to senior school?' is too narrow, because the answer will lack depth and analysis possibilities. Once you have worked out what defines a person as a

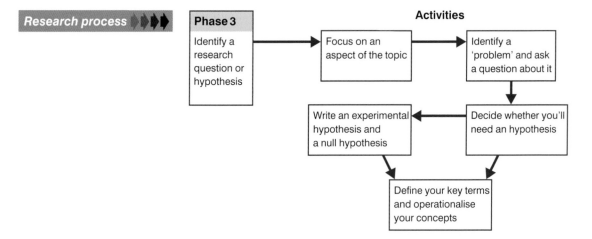

Figure 6.2 *Phase 3: Identifying a research question*

'physiotherapy student in England', and what counts as 'studying physiotherapy', the answer will be a simple number. The data won't really say anything about the experience of physiotherapy students and their mobility around the country in undertaking physiotherapy training. On the other hand, 'What's the experience of physiotherapy students training in England who are studying physiotherapy in the county where they went to school?' is too broad and open-ended for a small-scale study. The concept of 'experience' is too vague at the moment and is likely to be problematic. A researchable question lies somewhere between these two examples.

Should you use a research question or hypothesis?

You will need to produce a hypothesis or a research question to clearly focus your investigation. Your decision about which to use will depend on the type of research that you wish to do and the theoretical approach that you take.

Hypotheses

You may have decided to investigate your chosen topic because you have a 'hunch' about something or because you want to test an existing theory. In this case, it would be appropriate to use a *hypothesis*. This is a statement that makes a prediction (your 'hunch') about what you will find or what will happen: for example, 'Physiotherapy tutors are more likely to vote for the Labour party than the Conservative party in a general election'. A hypothesis is really a part of a bigger theory about what's believed to be true in the situation that you are investigating.

As a researcher, your task is to test the hypothesis (the prediction) by assessing whether the evidence supports or contradicts it. This is sometimes called a *deductive* approach. The researcher tries to deduce, or work out, whether there is evidence to support the hypothesis or 'hunch'. If your research evidence does not support the hypothesis (prediction), this might lead you to question and doubt the bigger theory. If the research evidence does support the hypothesis, it might strengthen your belief in the bigger theory. Because the evidence could possibly go either way (supporting or contradicting the hypothesis), two hypotheses are needed. Researchers who adopt this approach tend to use what are called an *experimental hypothesis* and a *null hypothesis*.

The experimental hypothesis is the predictive statement that you make: for example, 'Bottle-fed babies are usually heavier than breast-fed babies'. This hypothesis states that there will be a measurable difference between two situations because of the effect of independent variable(s). The independent variable is the factor (breast- or bottle-feeding) that the researcher thinks might influence change (weight of baby). However, because the evidence from a research study may not support the experimental hypothesis, researchers produce what's called a null hypothesis. This states that any change that occurs, or lack of change, in the situation is due to chance, or to some factor other than the independent variable.

Hypotheses can be *directional* or *non-directional*. If you predict that change will occur in a particular way (that something will increase or decrease), you will be making a directional hypothesis. If you simply predict that change will occur, without saying how it will occur, you will be using a non-directional hypothesis.

Can you develop a research question rather than a hypothesis?

It is not always necessary to use a hypothesis in a research investigation. For example, if you are going to do exploratory or descriptive, qualitative research using a naturalistic approach, you may simply want to gain a better understanding of the specific topic that you are investigating. In this case you would be better off with a research question to guide your work, but you won't need to make any predictions about what you will find. Researchers who begin with a general question are said to adopt an *inductive approach*: that is, they tend to get very involved in an area and try to work out the sense in the data that they collect. Inductive research works from evidence towards theory – in contrast to deductive research, which begins with the theory and tests it against the evidence.

Table 6.2 **Students' ideas for health and social care research projects**		
Research topic	**Question or hypothesis**	**Main methodology**
Surrogate pregnancy	Under what circumstances is surrogacy acceptable?	Questionnaire survey
Water birth	What do women think about water births?	Questionnaire survey and interviews
Informal care	How satisfied are informal carers with their access to community physiotherapy?	Questionnaires and interviews
Health promotion	How effective are current media in promoting healthy eating?	Questionnaires and interviews
Alzheimer's disease	Is it possible to care for people with Alzheimer's disease without using drugs?	Interviews and secondary data review
Cannabis	Should cannabis be legalised for medicinal purposes?	Questionnaires and interviews
Health-care roles	What are occupational therapists' attitudes towards OT assistants/aids?	Questionnaires and interviews
Suicide	Young people under 25 are less likely to disapprove of suicide than people over the age of 50	In-depth interviews
Gay relationships	Health-care workers are more likely to disapprove of gay relationships between members of their own sex than between two members of the opposite sex	Questionnaires Photograph response test
Premature birth	Has the survival rate of premature babies changed over the last 20 years?	Analysis of statistics and treatment
Male carers	What do women think of male midwives?	Questionnaires and interviews
Smoking	What factors influence doctors to smoke?	Questionnaires and interviews
Children's play	Is there a gender-related pattern to play in the waiting area of the children's outpatients department?	Observations

Operational concepts and identifying variables

Whatever the research question or hypothesis that you come up with, it is highly likely that it will contain a number of terms that will need to be clarified and explained very clearly as part of your project preparation. Look at the following research question:

What are occupational therapists' attitudes towards OT helpers/assistants?

You will notice that 'occupational therapists' and 'OT helpers/assistants' are key terms in the question. Both these terms need to be defined by the researcher and are used to identify a particular type or group of people. But what indicators should be used to classify a person as an 'occupational therapist' or an 'OT assistant'? Is it the amount of training they have received, is it about their title, is about what they do? Similarly, what is meant by 'attitudes'? This is a concept (an idea) that describes a predisposition to think and behave in either a positive or negative way, but how should the researcher (and the readers of the research report) distinguish attitudes? Before s/he can go any further, the researcher has to decide what indicates occupational therapist and OT assistant status and what the term 'attitude' includes.

Look at the question again. We still haven't 'operationalised' the key concept or idea that we are studying. The concept that we are actually trying to measure is 'attitude'. As researchers, we have to decide how to measure 'attitude'. Maybe we could measure it through a questionnaire that gives attitudinal ratings, or perhaps you could observe behaviours of occupational therapists towards OT assistants or give the occupational therapists some clinical scenarios and interview them about their thoughts and behaviours about the clinical situation. There are lots of potential indicators of 'attitude' that could be used, each with its own strengths and weaknesses. As a researcher, you have to choose the best indicator(s), the ones that you feel are most useful. When you have clearly defined all the terms (we could also call them variables) in your research question or hypothesis, you will have operationalised your concepts!

In the example we are using, this would mean operationalising 'occupational therapists' (e.g. registered occupational therapists working in acute hospitals). Also operationalising 'OT assistants' (e.g. staff working in acute hospital settings who are employed to

Keywords

Operational definition
One in which all terms have
been defined by the steps
(or operations) used to
measure them – this helps
eliminate confusion in
meaning and any possible
ambiguity in communication

deliver occupational therapy under the supervision of a registered
occupational therapist). Even although the meanings of some of
these terms might seem obvious, you can see through the examples
how important it is to define precisely how they will be used in
your investigation.

The readers of your research report will expect you to explain and
justify the ways in which you operationalise your concepts. When you
read research reports you should also try to find out how the key
concepts have been operationalised and comment on the adequacy of
the way in which this has been done.

Reflective activity

Identifying and operationalising concepts

Look at this research question:

Do young women think that water birth is an acceptable way to deliver a baby?

Now try to:

- Define the key terms
- Identify possible indicators of the key research concept that will help you
  to operationalise it.

You might like to write out your own research question or hypothesis,
have a go at defining the key terms and then think about how you could
operationalise the key research concepts.

Rapid recap

Check your progress so far by working through each of the following questions.

1. Are you going to use a hypothesis, a research question or both?
2. What's your general research question?
3. Do you have a null hypothesis as well as an experimental hypothesis,
   or is this not necessary?
4. Which terms in the research question do you have to define?
5. How have you operationalised the concepts that you are going to research?

If you have other questions, doubts about or problems relating to identifying
a research question or hypothesis and you are doing a research study
in your course, you should talk them through with your tutor or supervisor
at an early opportunity.

Reference

Langley, P. (1993) *Managing Sociology Coursework.* Connect Publications, Lewes, Sussex.

Further reading

Cormack, D. and Benton, D. (1996) Asking the research question, in: *The Research Process in Nursing* (eds W. Chenitz and J. Swanson). Addison-Wesley, Menlo Park, CA, pp. 102–120.

Using background literature in research

'Reviewing the field', as it is often called, is an essential task during the planning and preparation stage of a research investigation. What it means is that the researcher needs to find and review relevant information and previous work done by others on their chosen topic. Professional and academic researchers talk about 'doing a literature review' and spend a lot of their time and energy tracking down and reviewing research literature. In practice, they use specialist, well-equipped academic libraries to identify research papers and books on their chosen topic that have been published throughout the world. Then they review them and summarise the useful bits. Before we consider what these might be, we need to briefly consider the purpose of searching for and using background information.

Research process ▶▶▶

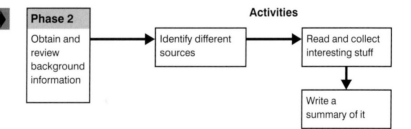

Figure 7.1 *Phase 2: Obtaining and reviewing background information*

Why obtain background information?

There are three main reasons for obtaining and reviewing background information on the chosen research topic.

It helps to clarify the research problem

In order to obtain background information, researchers need to have a good idea of the kind of thing that they are looking for. The process of searching through and reviewing information sources helps to focus the research idea more clearly.

It also helps in the decisions regarding development of the methodology

Finding examples of previous research investigations on the general area – or even the precise problem to be studied – gives a very good idea of how the area can be investigated. Previous studies can help researchers to develop their own approach, research design and data collection methods. Sometimes it is appropriate to try something different from the work of previous researchers, but there may also be very good reasons for replicating previously used methods. One of the key outcomes of the background information review should be that it assists in explaining and defending the decisions made regarding your investigation.

It should improve understanding about the research topic

Developing a broader and deeper understanding of the topic area of the research is probably the most important reason for obtaining and reviewing background information. Researchers should know about

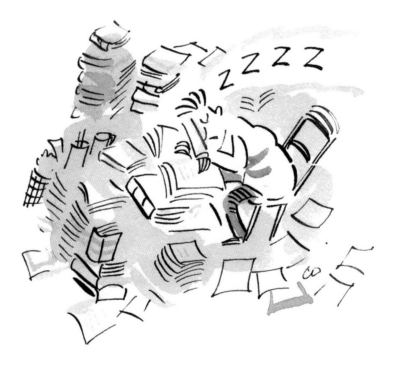

Be selective about the literature that you choose to review or your project will never get past this stage

the theories and evidence that currently exist in the topic area. This will enable them to understand where their own research investigation fits into the area. The conventional search of background information, or 'literature review' as it is termed in the research process, may not be as comprehensive in an exploratory study, as the researcher may want to avoid going in with preconceived ideas about the subject under investigation (Strauss and Corbin 1998). In most student health-care research studies, however, you would be advised to undertake a literature review to help you clarify the research problem, develop your methodology and improve your understanding of the research topic.

The extent of the literature search should largely be determined by the scope of the topic area and the time available to undertake the research. It is useful to set parameters as to how broad the background reading will be, otherwise too much time can be spent on this stage and the research findings will not be delivered on time.

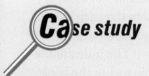 **Case study**

Lesley's research project

Lesley has decided to investigate the area of smoking cessation. She spent some time with the smoking cessation nurse specialist when on placement and noticed that she was involved in individual and group health promotion activities trying to assist people in stopping their smoking. She is struggling to decide the parameters of her literature review.

Reflective activity

Reflect on the problem that Lesley faces and consider the following issues that will help to resolve her dilemma:

- Should she restrict her literature search to British sources?
- How far back chronologically should she research?
- Should she look only at literature sources that refer to smoking cessation rather than more broadly at health promotion?
- Should she look at literature on the role of the nurse specialist?
- Should she explore literature regarding nicotine replacement therapy?
- Should she get policy documents from government sources on smoking cessation?

Sources for background information

'How do you search for background information?' The answer to this question ultimately depends on the researcher's ability to obtain access to different types of information resource. In theory, a number of potential resources are typically available, and these include the following.

Textbooks

In education institutes there are a wide variety of textbooks. Textbooks provide summaries of, and commentaries on, theories and pieces of research, and aim to be as accessible as possible. They may also include examples of statistics, quotes or extracts from important or hard-to-find documents.

A limitation of textbooks as a source of background information is that they provide only *secondary data*. These are in the form of second-hand accounts of research studies or explanations of theories, and are usually fairly brief. Textbooks may be useful in the early stages of a literature search, as the researcher tries to get some idea of the kinds of research that have been done on the subject. The index of the textbook can be used to identify coverage of the topic within the book. Care needs to be taken in making sure that the bibliography section is referred to, and details kept so that the original source of the information is noted. This kind of detail is needed in the final write-up so that all the sources used to complete the project are adequately referenced. Reference details can also point towards other specialist topic books, which may or may not be primary sources but are likely to have more detail on the topic than a textbook can give.

Topic books

A subject or keyword search on the computerised catalogue at the library produces a list of book titles on the chosen topic. These more specialist topic books can be a good source of detail and add depth to the background information. The researcher has to work at identifying and summarising the interesting and relevant bits of information.

As with textbooks, a useful way of identifying other publications on a similar subject is the bibliography at the back of the book, and this approach can also be used when reading journal articles.

Journals

Professional and academic researchers publish accounts of their research studies and their findings in specialist research journals. These can be very useful to obtain and some online versions also provide full text reports on areas of interest. Very specialist research journals may not be available in the education institute library and there will be a wait while they are obtained. It is therefore crucial that the researcher starts to collect background information/literature at an early stage in the project.

Magazines and newspapers

Magazine and newspaper stories – particularly in the form of survey findings or case studies – may provide some useful and accessible background information. The researcher needs to think carefully about the validity of the information found in magazines and newspapers. However, it does give an indication of media and public interest in the issue examined. Magazines, and many newspapers, are primarily aiming to entertain their readers rather than to add anything significant to their knowledge and understanding of a subject. Many academic researchers write for specialist magazines and are more likely than journalists to give reliable and valid information on specialist subjects.

Newspapers are often a good source of current information on a subject. The broadsheets (large-format newspapers) tend to be more reliable and impartial than the tabloid newspapers (those with a smaller page size) as a source of research data and balanced reporting. It is helpful to look for news articles written by established researchers and authors on the area of research interest.

CD-ROMs

CD-ROMs are a very popular way of searching for information because they are quick and easy to use. Many of the CD-ROM encyclopedias do have useful summaries of social science, psychology and health-related topics, but this coverage is always limited. Further information is always required, and it is unlikely that up-to-date statistics or accounts of research studies will be found on CD-ROMs.

The Internet

The Internet is very popular with students and other first-time researchers as a potential source of background information for their projects. While it has huge potential and is very convenient as a source of information, you need to be aware that research on the Internet is very different from traditional library research. A *search engine*, a program set up to guide the researcher through a mass of information to what is relevant, can be accessed through a 'key word' search. The search engine, however, does not discriminate between websites.

The books and journals found in libraries have nearly always been through a thorough review and evaluation process by subject experts before they are published. As a result, you can usually rely on the information in books and journals being reliable and objective. By contrast, you cannot rely on websites to be reliable sources of valid and objective information. Anyone can publish anything on the Internet. In some ways this can be thought of as a strength, but it is

---

Key points | **Top tips**

Researching on the Internet

- Make use of *both* library and online resources
- Cross-check any information obtained from the Internet with authoritative library resources
- Evaluate the Internet sites that you use. Ask the following questions:
  - Can you identify the author(s) of the web pages or websites?
  - Are the author(s) well known in the area that you are researching?
  - Do the authors give their credentials and their reasons for publishing the information?
  - Is the site linked to other authoritative and reputable sites?
  - Where did the author(s) gather their information from?
  - Is the information based on original research or secondary sources?
  - When was the information published? (Many sites are never updated or properly maintained)
  - Is the information academic in nature (produced by researchers), popular (produced for the general public), governmental or commercial (produced by a business for commercial reasons)?
  - Does the information express an opinion or claim to be factual? How does the information compare with what you already know? Does it add anything to your understanding of the topic?
- Keep a detailed record of the sites that you access and the sources of the information that you use. It is best to bookmark the good sites that you use and organise them in a directory so that you will be able to find them again. Reference the sites that you use in your final report.

also an important weakness for information accessed in this way by a researcher. Because there is usually no review or screening of the information, care has to be taken when doing a research literature search online.

Organisations

Many commercial, voluntary and statutory organisations conduct research studies that they then publish. If you wish to explore this possible source of information, you will need to identify organisations that operate, or have an interest, in the area that you are studying. It is worth contacting relevant organisations in order to obtain their publications list. This may reveal the existence of books, booklets, websites and reports that can be used to deepen understanding of the research topic. Often, luckily, the information is free.

The reliability and validity of any information that you obtain is important. With this in mind, it is important to note that organisations do not often do 'disinterested' research. They usually have a particular set of objectives or goals in mind and do research to further the causes that they believe in. As such, objectivity can be an issue. To assess whether the information found is objective, it is best to use a variety of sources and to cross-check between them. This helps in making judgements about the reliability of each source and the validity of the background information collected.

There are a range of health, medicine and social care specific databases that can be accessed through the Internet. These include OVID (http://gateway.ovid.com/) and Medline (http://www.ncbi.nih.gov/entrez/query.fcgi). The literature references that can be obtained through these sources are peer-reviewed. Following an initial reading of the abstract supplied with each reference, you should be able to identify how useful this referenced article is to your research project. If you have to undertake a research study your higher education institution will be able to advise you about the most appropriate sources for the study you are undertaking. Many tutors and librarians will also provide advice and guidance on how to go about accessing information from these sources.

Keeping track of sources used as background information

As a conscientious and enthusiastic researcher, you should seek out and review numerous pieces of background information from various sources. It is important that you keep a record of all the different sources that you have reviewed and read. If you do not, you will have to go back and retrace your sources at the end of the project. This can be very time-consuming and frustrating and, with a little advance planning, can be avoided.

Dealing with the information

Once sufficient background information has been obtained it will need to be summarised. Basically this involves writing an overview of the main issues, theories and research findings about the area of interest. This needs to be done with the proposed topic and research question in mind. Compiling a literature review summary can take some time to complete because usually there is a large amount of information to deal with. Time should be taken to write in a considered, structured format that outlines the main themes and summarises these while avoiding too much detail. The overview should focus the reader's attention on key points and end up by locating the choice of research topic within the overall area. The literature review should also critique the literature, as some sources will be more valid than others. The literature review should be organised into linked sections. The progression through the literature should broadly match the sections suggested by the following statements:

- This is what the topic is about
- This is what people think or have found so far
- This is a critique of the literature already available
- These are the main issues
- This is the aspect of the topic that my research is going to address

When you have to do a literature review your research supervisor or tutor will tell you how long your background information/literature review ought to be. You should know the minimum and maximum word counts before you begin, so that you can avoid writing too little – or, more likely, too much.

Reflective activity

Considering background information issues

- Think back to your experience of a recent clinical placement area. Try to identify an incident that occurred during the placement that stands out in your memory as significant.
- Write a few descriptive sentences about the incident.
- Examine the incident again. Identify a researchable topic or issue within it on which you could conduct a small-scale study.
- Write down your responses to each of the prompts below to demonstrate that you have thought through the various aspects involved in obtaining and reviewing background information on it.
  - Where can you get your background information from?
  - Have you identified a range of different sources?
  - What kinds of information are you looking for?
  - What parameters would you set for the literature search?
  - What structure would you give to the literature?
  - How would you relate the background information to your research idea?

Rapid recap

Check your progress so far by working through each of the following questions.

1. Give two reasons for undertaking a background literature review before starting a research study.
2. Identify as many possible sources for background literature that a researcher could access.

If you have difficulty with either of the questions, read through the section again to refresh your understanding before moving on.

Reference

Strauss, A and Corbin, J (1998) *Basics of qualitative research: Techniques and procedures for developing grounded theory,* 2nd ed., Sage, Thousand Oaks, California.

Further reading

Clarke, R. and Croft, P. (1998) *Critical Reading for the Reflective Practitioner: A guide for primary care*. Butterworth-Heinemann, Oxford.

Reading and evaluating published research

Keywords

Research critique

To carefully read a piece of research and appraise yourself of its strengths and limitations. The practitioner who is not technically ready to undertake their own research can be perfectly competent to evaluate the work of others. This evaluation needs to be constructive, penetrating and as value-free as possible

What is a critical evaluation?

As a student health-care practitioner, you may not be required to do a small-scale research study in your course but you will at some point be required to read and evaluate a piece of published research. You could also be asked to undertake a literature review. This involves critically evaluating a range of published research on a topic. An evaluation involves making a judgement about the relative strengths and weaknesses or overall value of something.

Critical evaluation skills allow an individual or a group to assess the worth of a research article or report by looking carefully at all the parts of the study. Any of the terms 'critical appraisal', 'critical evaluation' or '**research critique**' can be used to describe the process of systematically and logically reading a research report and giving a balanced opinion on it.

Just because the term 'critical' is used it does not mean that the research should be read in a negative, 'fault-finding' way. However, it does mean that the research should be read carefully and assessed objectively. Health-care practitioners who want to give evidence-based care need to have the skills to critically evaluate other people's research reports. A clear knowledge and understanding of the research process is needed to provide a critical evaluation of a research paper.

How can you tell if a report is a research paper or an article?

Sometimes it can be difficult to decide whether the research report you are reading is an original piece of research or a literature review, a case study, a discussion paper or some other type of report or article.

The easiest way of deciding whether you have got a research paper is to read the summary or abstract that outlines the content of the report and find sections within it that talk about the aims of the research, the sample that was studied and the methods of collecting data.

If you are able to choose a published paper to review, you should choose a paper from a recognised academic or professional journal that specialises in publishing research papers. Some professional journals that provide reports of research studies do not actually publish whole research papers. For example, although the *Health Service Journal* contains a popular summary of the latest research within its articles, these do not give the full outline of the research methods used and would not be appropriate for your review. You would still need to go to the original published research paper to obtain this detailed information.

When you first start to evaluate research studies in the way we are about to outline it can seem really time-consuming as there are lots of questions and points to consider. However, you will speed up as you practise these skills and the stages become more familiar to you.

ReflectReflective activity

Reading a research report 'normally'

Find a research article that you think is interesting. Read it as you would normally do and jot down the key pieces of information as you discover them.

If someone were to ask you 'Is that article any good?', what would you say to them? Jot this down. Keep your notes, as later on you will be able to compare what you found out from reading the research article 'normally' to what you find when doing a critical evaluation of it.

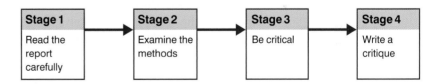

Stage 1	Stage 2	Stage 3	Stage 4
Read the report carefully	Examine the methods	Be critical	Write a critique

Figure 8.1 *The four stages of critical evaluation*

Stage 1: Reading a research report critically

The first thing to do in a critical evaluation is to find out what the research report actually says. Start with the title and the abstract or summary, if the report has one. This will give you an overview of what the paper is about and the kind of conclusions that are reached.

During reading you should first look for answers to the following preliminary questions:

- What is the title of the report?
- Who did the research? Was he or she qualified to carry out this type of work? Was this the first piece of research the investigator carried out?
- What is the study about? Is there an abstract or summary? Does the title of the report accurately reflect the problem studied?
- Why was it done? Was the purpose of the study worthwhile?
- Where was it published? What assessment can be made from the way the study is presented as to its quality and to its relevance to your practice?
- Who funded the research? Did the researcher(s) have adequate support and resources?

Who did the research? When you ask these questions you start to think about the credentials (qualifications and experience) of the researcher(s). The researcher may have research-specific qualifications – e.g. PhD, research doctorate – or have done research as part of their degree. Their current employment will show whether they are in a full-time research post (as, for example, a research fellow) or have undertaken their research as part of their professional practice. Your questions will also find out whether the research was carried out in your own country, as this could have a bearing on how relevant it is to your practice. If the research was about emergency nursing in America, this may take a very different form from accident and emergency nursing in the UK and this needs to be kept in mind when reviewing the paper.

What is the study about? The title may not fully explain the area covered in the research, even though research titles are often quite long, but you should be able to work out clearly from the abstract and initial reading what the research problem is –'What question was the researcher trying to answer?' Perhaps s/he was trying to explore an issue or demonstrate a link between particular variables. There will be some unknown area on which the research is trying to cast some light. You need to identify it. You should try to identify the aims and objectives of the investigation. How this study links with existing theory, knowledge and previous research should be clearly explained.

Why was it done? The research article should contain a justification for why the research was undertaken. You should also on this first careful reading be aware of the main findings from the research. Your decision as to whether the research was worthwhile depends partly on how much it relates to your own interests and partly how it relates to existing research.

Where was it published? There are an increasing number of research journals that publish health and social care literature and these vary greatly in their quality, especially in the standards they use to accept papers for publication. Before research is published in a journal, it has usually gone through a process of scrutiny and review. Editors will take a look at potentially suitable articles and will send these to a panel of expert reviewers to judge the quality of the research and how appropriate it is for that particular journal. Even if the journal that the research comes from has a reputation for carefully reviewing papers before accepting them for publication, you still need to carefully evaluate the research paper, answering the questions outlined in this chapter.

The publication date of the study may be easy to find out, but if you have not been able to find out you can assume that there was a gap between writing and publishing. This can even be a gap of more than 2 years. This may not always matter, but in areas where practice is changing quickly the information may be out of date.

Who funded the research? If the research has not been externally funded and the researcher has carried out the research within his/her everyday professional practice, this may have limited its scale. If the research study has external funding, for instance by drug manufacturers, the interests of those funding it may have influenced the published results.

At the start of writing up your critical evaluation you will need to summarise the article. Basically, you need to provide a brief descriptive account of what the research was about, who did the research, how it was done and what was found. Try to be clear, precise and unambiguous in the way in which you report on the study.

Reflect*Reflective activity*

Critically evaluating a research report (Stage 1)

Using the same research article you used in the last reflective activity, work your way through the preliminary questions that form Stage 1 of the critical evaluation process.

Compare the notes that you produce in response to the structured, basic set of critical questions with your jottings from the first 'normal' reading of the research paper. You should notice that the 'normal' jottings are less descriptive and that they show a less questioning attitude to what you have read than the notes produced from your second, more critical, reading.

Stage 2: Examine the methods

You should now know the questions and the answers resulting from the research investigation that you are reading about. The next stage is to examine the methods used. You need to find out what the researcher did and how s/he did it. It is best to read the report in a way that enables you to answer the questions that you want to ask rather than reading it from beginning to end in a conventional manner. There is a common format to research reports. The second step of a critical evaluation involves breaking up the article into specific sections. The writer of the article has often made this easier by writing the report using section headings such as:

- Introduction and background to the study
- Review of the literature
- Research design and approach
- Sampling strategy and selection of subjects
- Data collection
- Data analysis and results
- Ethical considerations
- Discussion.

Look at each of these sections in turn and make notes in response to the questions that are identified for each section. This will enable you to understand the decisions made by the researcher and will help you to identify the strengths and weaknesses of the study. If you come across terms or phrases that you do not understand you will need to look them up before carrying on. If you do not do this you may end up making a judgement about something you do not fully understand.

Introduction and background to the study

- Is the problem or area of research clearly explained and justified?
- Is the background to the research logically presented?
- Are the limitations of the study acknowledged?

The decisions that have to be made during the research process mean that there will always be limitations to a research study and the researcher should be open and honest about these.

Review of the literature

- Was an up-to-date and relevant review of previous work included?
- Was the literature search adequate?

This section may be quite short within an article compared to a full research report, but you should still be able to get a sense of whether major studies have been looked at.

Research design and approach

- If theoretical frameworks are used, are these explained and linked to the research design?
- Are the research questions clearly expressed?
- Are definitions given, and are they clear and concise?
- What was the research strategy – a survey, an experiment, a case study, an observation or something else?
- Is the research design suitable for the research problem?

Sometimes theory can be referred to in a research study but appears to have little linkage to it. You need to look at whether the research design and approach is, in your opinion, the best solution to the research question.

Sampling strategy and selection of subjects

- Who, or what population, was the study about?
- How was sampling carried out – how many in the sample?
- Was the sampling method adequate?
- Are there any potential sampling biases?

The design of the study should aim to minimise bias in the recruitment of subjects. If the researcher fails to provide important bits of information (such as how many people actually returned the questionnaire sent to them) you should be suspicious. You should not just assume that the researcher simply forgot to mention this detail.

Data collection

- What data were collected?
- What instruments or tools were used?
- Were the instruments used valid and reliable?
- Under what circumstances were the data collected?
- Was a pilot study conducted to establish and refine the methods used?

If a research tool has been designed specifically for the study, an account of the process of how the tool was developed and tested should be included in the report.

Data analysis and results

- Is the way the data are organised and analysed adequate?
- If it is a quantitative study are the statistics correctly performed?
- Are the tables and graphs properly labelled?
- If it is a qualitative study are major 'themes' identified, and is there a description of how the data were analysed and validity checked?
- What were the main results of the study?

The researcher should keep to the data and explain how any conclusions made are based on the evidence. You should look carefully for any evidence of bias in the interpretation of the results.

Ethical considerations

- Does the researcher appear to have acted in a professional manner throughout the research?
- Was permission to undertake the research given by a Research Ethics Committee?

There are ethical issues in all research, and the researcher should have considered and included them in the report. Sometimes this is done in a separate section, or ethical issues may be integrated throughout the report.

Discussion

- Is the discussion clearly separate from the actual findings?
- Are the recommendations for practice, education, management or policy development related appropriately to the research?

In this section the researcher draws the study together and makes recommendations, including areas for further research. It is here that the findings of the study are discussed, relating back to the literature review and the background information. They may also indicate limitations and weaknesses of the study in this section.

This seems like a lot of questions in Stage 2 but as you get used to reading research in this critical way you will need to refer to them less and less. The difficulty you have had in reading the article or report may be because it is not clearly written, has unnecessary jargon, is not logically structured or the references are not consistent or accurate. Within your critical evaluation you can comment on the overall presentation of the research as well.

Stage 3: Being critical

Most evaluations require you to be critical. If you have asked all the questions included you should be able to be critical. This is not an opportunity to say that everything about the study was awful – or an invitation to criticise the researcher in any personal sense. A critical evaluation requires you to identify the relative strengths and weaknesses of the methods used in the study, and to assess the findings and conclusions in the light of the methods used to obtain them. Work your way through the findings and match them up to the conclusions. Check that each of the conclusions is supported by the researcher's evidence. You may want to raise doubts about the validity of some findings in the light of the methods used to collect it. You will then have to decide whether the conclusions still hold, despite the weaknesses that you see in the evidence.

Stage 4: Write a critique

A critique is a considered, argued but balanced appraisal of the research report. Approach it in an objective and structured way.

- Begin with a balanced account of the research study.
- Next, identify and discuss the strengths of the researcher's approach.
- Move on to identify any parts of the original questions or objectives that the research does not seem to address.
- You might then discuss the logic of the argument(s) that the researcher puts forward, particularly if there are contradictions or problems with them.
- Now you are left with the conclusions. Consider the areas in which the evidence for the conclusions is either strong or weak. You may want to comment on the extent to which the methods used to obtain the data limit the generalisation or validity of the conclusions.

- Towards the end of your critique you will need to look at ethical issues. Appraise the extent to which the researcher protected or placed participants 'at risk', and assess the adequacy of the confidentiality procedures and the efforts made to avoid introducing bias.

- Finally, you will need to arrive at a conclusion about the research study that you are appraising. You will need to identify what has – and what hasn't – been shown to be true, and what you feel the overall strengths and weaknesses of the investigation were.

Why spend so long in reading one piece of research?

If you compared your simple, 'normal' reading of an article to your second critical reading you should have started to answer this question. Although evaluating a research study takes a considerable amount of time it is really important to gain these skills. Previously in the book the importance of evidence-based practice has been discussed. If a health-care practitioner cannot evaluate research he/she might change their practice after reading a research article which has serious flaws. This could have poor outcomes for the patient whose care has been changed in response to this research study.

When you first undertake research evaluation you will need to refer to the stages and questions outlined in this chapter but as you do this more frequently you will need to refer to this framework less often. You probably already have a good idea of some of the things you will consider when you next read some research. It is also useful, if you are doing your own research study, to ask the same questions of your study as it will help you to identify limitations and to be honest in your research report about these.

Reflective activity

Using the research article you obtained for the previous activity in this section complete the Research Critique Checklist and add your comments to the research report critique form and then compare those made on your first time of reading the article.

Checklist for a Research Critique

Is there a clearly formulated hypothesis or research question? ☐

Is the focus of the study clearly explained? ☐

Are the researchers credible to undertake this research? ☐

Is there a suitable review of supporting research literature? ☐

Is the supporting theoretical literature linked to the research effectively? ☐

Is the research approach suitable for the research question/hypothesis? ☐

Have the research participants been selected appropriately? ☐

Has the researcher used quality control measures to ensure reliability of data? ☐

Has the researcher used quality control measures to ensure validity of data? ☐

Has the data been analysed appropriately? ☐

Have the potential biases been minimised? ☐

Are the main results of the study clear? ☐

Have ethical considerations been handled properly? ☐

Has the research provided credible and significant results? ☐

Has the research demonstrated generalisability of the research? ☐

Has the discussion and recommendations been developed from the findings? ☐

Has the research demonstrated any obvious application to patient or clinical care? ☐

Has the research been presented and disseminated in a suitable way? ☐

Table 8.1 **Research report critique (note strengths and weaknesses for each section)**	
Title of study	
Authors	
Date of study	Date of publication
Aim of study	
Research question (hypotheses)	
Background information and literature review	
Sample and sample size	
Method of study and research tools used	
Analysis and findings	
Ethical issues	
Discussion and conclusion	

~~RRRRR~~Rapid recap

Check your progress so far by working through each of the following questions.

1. What does the term critical evaluation mean?
2. What are the four main stages in constructing a research critique?
3. Why is having the ability to critique research a useful skill for health-care practitioners?

If you have difficulty with more than one of the questions, read through the section again to refresh your understanding before moving on.

Further reading

Abreu, B., Peloquin, S. and Ottenbacher, K. (1998) Competence in scientific inquiry and research. *American Journal of Occupational Therapy*, **52**, 751–759.

Greenhalgh, T. and Taylor, R. (1997) How to read a research paper: papers that go beyond numbers (qualitative research). *British Medical Journal*, **315**, 740–743.

9 Research strategies

Learning outcomes

By the end of this chapter you should be able to:

- Discuss the main types of research strategy
- Appreciate the importance of decisions regarding sampling
- Identify the advantages and disadvantages of using a survey, experimental, case study and action research strategy.

Deciding on a research strategy

Once you have decided on the topic or practice area that you wish to research, and have focused on an aspect of it by writing a research question – and perhaps a hypothesis – you will need to do some practical planning. In particular, you will need to decide how to actually approach and structure your investigation. In short, you need to choose a research strategy and decide on a research design. Both of these things must fit your research question and/or hypothesis.

Choosing a research design

A research design is a general plan of how the research investigation will be run and organised. Questions need to be answered. For example, will there be one data collection period or will data be collected before and then after some event (such as an activity or test)? Will data collection be about something that has happened in the past (for example, inpatients who have lost more than a kilogram in weight during their admission to the hospital)? Is a comparison of data from two different time periods required (for example, 'this month' compared to 'the same month last year')? The various research design options available are outlined and discussed in the next chapter.

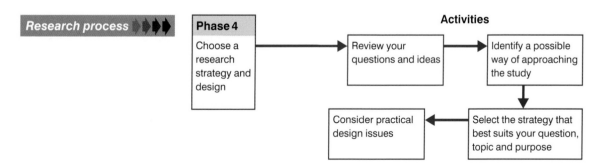

Figure 9.1 *Phase 4: Choosing a research strategy and design*

Choosing a research strategy

In general terms, a research strategy is an overall methodology. It is a decision about the data collection tactics to be used. For a small-scale piece of project research, the choice might be made between adopting a survey approach, doing an experiment, carrying out a case study or conducting a piece of action research.

A research strategy is different from a data collection method. The research strategy defines the general approach to the research investigation. The data collection methods that are used are not predetermined by the choice of research strategy. Whatever strategy is chosen, it is generally possible to use a variety of different data collection methods. For example, you could use interviews, questionnaires or observation to obtain data in either a piece of action research or a survey.

Think of a research strategy as a type of holiday. You can probably imagine lots of different types of holiday (beach holidays, skiing holidays and city breaks, for example). Now think of data collection methods as ways of getting to your holiday destination (flying, driving, taking a ferry or walking, for example). You could use most of these methods to go on any type of holiday, but you would probably choose the most efficient. The same applies to data collection methods. Some methods, such as questionnaires, are ideal for conducting a survey, but you could also survey people's views by conducting interviews, even though it would probably be a less efficient method of collecting similar data.

The strategic decisions about how to carry out your research investigation may be influenced by a number of factors. For example:

- You may want to replicate the methods used in studies and reports that you have read about, where the research topic is similar to your own
- You may want to adopt a particular theoretical approach (for example, naturalistic research) or data collection method (for example, questionnaires)
- You will need to take account of practical factors, such as time and money – you cannot do a large-scale postal survey unless you can afford the postage charges!
- You will also need to take into account the difficulty of gaining access to important sources of data – an investigation into the social life of drug misusers might prove a bit too hazardous and difficult for this reason.

You should make an assessment of the strengths and limitations of the different strategy options open to you. If you are doing a small-scale research project you will need to do this in relation to your proposed research project and choose the one that is most appropriate to your project's objectives. The choice of research strategy will probably be made at an early stage in the life of a project.

When choosing a strategy the time available to complete the project needs to be taken into account. Decisions made at the start of the research project need to be made carefully because, if things do not seem to be working out, it is unlikely that there will be enough time to start again and adopt a different strategy. In the next section various strategy options will be considered.

Surveys

Researchers who conduct surveys take a broad, systematic view of a topic at a specific moment in time and collect empirical data (the observed 'facts') on it. Survey researchers go for breadth, incorporating data as inclusively as possible, in an attempt to 'bring things up to date' on their chosen subject.

It is possible to do a survey using questionnaires, interviews or observational methods, or by reviewing documents. However, most

Table 9.1 **The advantages and limitations of surveys**

Survey approach	Advantages	Limitations
Postal questionnaire survey	● Saves on interviewing time ● Can reach a large number of people easily ● Respondents can think about their answers to the questionnaire	● Response rates are often low ● You do not know who actually fills in the questionnaire ● Can be expensive
Face-to-face interview	● Response rate high ● The interviewer can clarify questions ● The interviewer can probe replies to get the full answers	● Time-consuming ● The interviewer may bias or influence respondents' answers
Telephone survey	● Convenient and quick ● The interviewer can clarify questions and probe answers	● Can be expensive ● You do not know who is answering ● People may not tell the truth, and you cannot see their non-verbal behaviour to assess this

people associate surveys with questionnaires and interviews as the main data collection tools. The choice of data collection method tends to depend on how the survey is conducted and the topic in question. Researchers who use questionnaires and interviews typically conduct their surveys by post, over the telephone and in face-to-face personal situations. The advantages and limitations of each of these ways of conducting a survey are outlined in Table 9.1.

The survey population and sampling

Choosing to adopt a survey strategy in a research investigation requires the researcher to identify their survey population and then select a sample from it. A *population* is the whole class of people or things that are being investigated.

Table 9.2 **What does a population consist of?**	
Focus of the survey	**Who are the population?**
Student attendance records on the last Friday before Christmas in higher education colleges and universities in Birmingham	All attendance registers in higher education colleges and universities in Birmingham on the last Friday before Christmas
Reasons why people attend Accident and Emergency Departments in London hospitals on a Friday night in August	All Accident and Emergency records of clients treated in London hospitals on Fridays nights in August
Social class of people in Glasgow who attended an osteopath for treatment during the last year	All people who have attended an osteopath in Glasgow in the last year and have had their social details recorded on the client records

As you can see, the population may – or, in the case of students attending lectures before Christmas, may not – consist of a large number of people or things. It is often impossible to distribute a questionnaire to, or conduct interviews with, every member of a research population. Even if the researcher were able to do this, the volume of work – as well as the expense and time – involved in tracking down every population member would probably lead to the investigation not being completed. The standard way out of these problems is to select a group of people or a number of items out of the whole population to represent it. This is known as *sampling*.

Choosing a research sample

Ideally, the sample should be representative of the whole population, so that your research conclusions can be generalised from it. However, in student research projects the sample does not necessarily have to be *precisely* representative of the population. Even so, any lack of representativeness should be acknowledged where it occurs. When undertaking some forms of research, such as a case study for example, there is less need to worry quite so much about it being representative.

The first key step in successfully selecting a sample is to ensure that you identify the research population clearly and specifically.

Example

An investigation of the alcohol consumption of student radiographers

Option 1   Radiography students

Option 2   Radiography students who consume alcohol

Option 3   Radiography students currently at your higher education institute who consume alcohol

Option 4   First year radiography students at your higher education institute who consume alcohol

---

In this example, the population is redefined four times. Each time, the definition becomes more precise. In option 1, the population would be all radiography students throughout the world. Option 2 narrows this down slightly to radiography students throughout the world who consume alcohol (there are probably some who do not). It would be impossible to interview or survey a representative sample of either of these large groups. The third option still leaves you with a fairly large group. It would be very difficult to contact and collect data from all individuals who are taking a radiography course at your college or university, unless you attend an institute with a small number of students who are doing radiography training courses. Option 4 is far more realistic and actually gives you a chance of completing your project!

There should be a list of first-year students who are currently studying at your institution. You could use this list to select a sample. The list of students is known as the *sampling frame*. Professional and academic researchers use a variety of different documents and databases as sampling frames.

Examples of sampling frames

- The telephone directory
- Outpatient clinic lists
- College/university enrolment lists and class registers
- Lists of employees/payrolls
- The electoral register
- Post Office address file
- Council tax register
- Professional registers
- Theatre lists

Researchers often try to make use of an existing sampling frame in their research project. Where no sampling frame currently exists for the intended population, you will have to compile one yourself. This can be time-consuming but may still be necessary. Alternatively, a convenience sample may have to be used or some very, very good reasons produced to explain why another unconventional sampling strategy is used. There is sometimes a temptation to try to use unorthodox sampling methods in an attempt to take a short cut or give a project something of an exotic edge. This needs to be resisted. Those reading the research are less likely to be impressed by a creative, but flawed, approach to sampling than by a clear, conscientious and well-executed use of more standard sampling procedures. It is best to learn how to use the orthodox approaches to population sampling before adapting or departing from them.

The generalisation of a survey's findings will depend on whether the sample is representative of the population as a whole. It is important to be aware that most samples are only representative in terms of particular, selected characteristics. If a sample needs to be representative of the research population in a particular way (for age or ethnicity, for example), the researcher has to ensure that the proportions of the selected characteristics in the sample match those in the population as a whole. The sample does not have to be representative of the population in other non-targeted ways. For example, it is unlikely that you would want to ensure an equal height match between the sample and the population in a study about sleeping patterns. In that study, height is likely to be irrelevant.

When defining a research population the researcher has to be very specific about the criteria needed for inclusion. As a student researcher you will also need to ensure that you identify a population to which you can gain access relatively easily. Remember that you will need to be able to make contact with a number of these people in a relatively short period of time. You will make the project much more difficult if you choose a population of people who are difficult to identify, track down or get time with.

How big should the sample be?

This is the question that all researchers doing surveys have to ask. Professional and academic researchers use relatively complicated statistical techniques to work out how big their samples should be, to make them representative of their research population and to allow them to generalise their findings.

In student research projects, size is less important. There are some general considerations to bear in mind, such as the following:

- Smaller samples are less likely to allow true representation of the diverse characteristics of the individuals who make up the population (unless the population is also very small!)
- Samples of fewer than 20 individuals won't usually generate enough data to allow the production of meaningful statistics
- Larger samples mean that there will be less opportunity to find out about each individual or case in the sample.

Practical considerations, such as how much time will be available, also affect decisions about sample size. First-time researchers should discuss the issue of sample size with their supervisor or research lecturer, who will be able to take into account the circumstances and nature of the investigation. As a very rough guide, a student survey that used a sample of between 30 and 60 individuals would generate enough data for analysis. Of course, getting 'enough data' also depends on how many questions are asked. If only two questions were asked, for instance, it is unlikely that there will be enough data: 15–20 questions would provide a more adequate and appropriate amount of data.

It is advisable to have a mixture of open and closed questions. 'Yes' and 'No' answers do not give much scope for analysis.

Choosing a method of sampling the population

There are basically two approaches to sampling a research population.

Probability methods

Probability methods give each member of the research population an equal chance (or probability) of being chosen as a part of the sample. For example, in our 'alcohol consumption' study we might select every second female radiography student from a list provided by your higher education institute. At the beginning, before we begin to make our selections, every student on the list has a 50% chance of being chosen at random, because we are choosing every second student. Chance will determine which particular members of the sample are selected. The purpose of random sampling is to reduce the potential for bias being introduced by the researcher.

Before you can use a probability sampling method, the researcher needs to be able to obtain, or produce, a complete list of all of the members of their research population. Remember that this list is known as the 'sampling frame'. The best known probability sampling method is *random sampling*.

One way of selecting members of the population at random is to arrange their names in a numbered list and then use a random-number table to pick numbers from the list. Alternatively, if there are only a relatively small number of names these can be written out separately and picked out at random from a 'hat'. Another alternative is to randomly choose one item to start with and then select every name at a given point onwards. For example, selection could begin at item six on the list and then the sample can be made up by selecting every fourth name.

Random samples can sometimes be non-representative. They can throw up, by chance, collections of people who are somehow not typical of the whole population. The risk of this happening can be overcome by using a second form of probability sampling, known as *stratified random sampling*. This involves identifying subgroups, or strata, within a population and then conducting a random sample of each of these subgroups to ensure that they are all represented in a sample. For example, in our 'alcohol consumption' study it might be appropriate to divide the list up. You could divide it according to age band, or even by ethnic group, or religious affiliation. Then when individuals are randomly selected from each stratum for the sample, this would arguably reduce the risk of obtaining an unrepresentative sample.

Purposive sampling methods

In purposive sampling methods the chance of a member of the research population being chosen is not equal and is sometimes unknown. This happens, for example, if you select all the first-year radiography students at your higher education institute. In this scenario, the first-year students have a 100% chance of being chosen for the sample, but the second-year students have a 0% chance. Alternatively, we might choose to select all radiography students who admit to drinking alcohol. We do not know how many there will be, and so do not know what the chance (probability) is of an individual being selected for the sample.

The best known form of purposive sampling is *quota sampling*. This allows researchers to control variables in their study without having a sampling frame. The researcher must identify the key criteria that all participants need to meet, and then approach people randomly to ask whether they meet these criteria and recruit a 'quota' of this group for research purposes. Once the quota for a particular group has been filled, the researcher won't seek or include any more people from that group.

Quota sampling is useful when the overall proportions of particular groups in the population are known. Quota sampling is not truly random sampling, as not everyone in a population has an equal chance of being selected. It is a form of sampling that is very useful to students who are carrying out relatively small research investigations in a short period of time. There is no need to have a definitive and complete sampling frame (unlike in stratified random sampling). Student researchers who have a good knowledge of the population that they

Sampling involves identifying and obtaining data from a limited number of people who meet specific criteria

seek to study can make an informed guess (but should acknowledge this!) to select quotas of individuals who are roughly representative of their research population. In a student research project, the quotas do not need to be in strict proportion to their incidence in the population but should be roughly so.

The choice of sampling method is usually determined by the need to keep the sampling process as simple as possible, by the likelihood of bias occurring in the sample and by the practicalities of what is actually possible. The researcher needs to choose the sampling method that best suits their project and which can be followed through and completed in the time available.

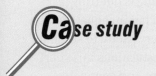

Case study

Example of research using a survey strategy

Roberts, J. and McKeown, K. (2001) Clinical governance for nurses: smoking cessation interventions. *Nursing Standard*, **15**, 33–36.

This was a postal survey of 800 clients, which received a response from 193. Of these 68% claimed to have been helped by smoking cessation services including; proactive telephone contact, carbon monoxide monitoring, 6-week course of nicotine replacement therapy and reading materials. At the time of the survey 36% of the respondents were no longer smoking.

Reflective activity

Undertaking a survey

Check your progress so far by working through each of the following questions. Write down your responses to each prompt to demonstrate that you have thought through the various aspects involved in using a survey strategy.

1. What data collection methods can be used to carry out a survey?
2. What would influence a decision to conduct a survey: face-to-face, over the phone or by post?
3. How does a researcher select a sample from within the population?
4. If no sampling frame exists what can the researcher do?

Experiments

Experiments are a very common and important research strategy. Like the other research strategies that we have covered so far, there are a variety of ways of collecting data in an experiment. The main characteristics of the experimental strategy relate to comparison and control, and seeking to find 'cause and effect' relationships.

Experiments tend to be the strategy of choice where biological, psychological or natural science phenomena are being investigated using a positivist approach. The vast majority of experiments in health-related research are laboratory experiments, or clinical trials, in which the effectiveness of medication and treatments for physical or psychiatric illnesses are investigated.

Health and social researchers are less likely than natural science researchers to use an experimental strategy. Where they do, they tend to conduct their investigations outside of a laboratory setting and run what are called 'field experiments'. An example might be an investigation into the reaction of psychiatrists to patients newly attending an outpatient psychiatric unit. In such an experiment the researcher might find that an actor dressed as a businessman received a longer consultation than the same actor dressed as a labourer, even although both claimed to have the same symptoms.

Characteristics of experiments

Experiments involve situations in which the researcher identifies two or more *variables* and then manipulates, or changes, one variable to see what effect, or consequence, this has on the other(s). These 'variables' are called the dependent and independent variables. The *dependent variable* is the thing or behaviour that the researcher wants to explain (e.g. 'anxiety levels'). The *independent variable* is the factor that the researcher thinks might influence the change (such as 'large spiders'). The independent variable is the thing that the researcher 'controls' in some way (such as showing people large spiders).

Researchers who use experiments typically wish to generate *quantitative* data and adopt a *positivist approach* to their research investigations. Experimental researchers place a lot of importance on establishing cause and effect relationships and carefully observe and measure what happens in the experimental situation. This is because they do not just want to know whether or not a relationship exists between two variables, they want to find out exactly how the relationship works.

Researchers who use experimental strategies make a considerable effort to isolate their experimental variables and reduce the influence of so-called *extraneous variables*. These are factors that may interfere with the relationship between the dependent and independent variables.

In experimental situations, researchers use a number of devices – such as control groups, placebos and 'blind' and 'double-blind' protocols – to promote and demonstrate the objectivity of their research.

A *control group* is a subgroup of research participants who are not experimented on. They are usually selected to match the qualities and characteristics of the experimental (tested) group. Findings obtained from the experimental group are then compared to those obtained from the control group (untested).

A *placebo* is an inert substance or phenomenon that has no known effect on the variable being tested. For example, instead of being given a real test drug in a clinical trial, some people may be given a 'sugar pill'. This looks the same as the real drug but does not contain the active ingredient. In clinical trials of medical drugs it is usual for half of the participants, the 'test' group, to be given the real drug (the independent variable), while the other half, the control group, receive the placebo. For the drug to be judged a success, the test group must experience significantly greater change in the dependent variable (whatever the intended action of the drug is – for example, mood change) than the placebo group. This would show that the independent variable (the real drug) was the factor that had a significant effect on the dependent variable. In other words, it would show that the drug worked!

Most clinical trials use a *blind protocol*. This means that the participants do not know whether they are receiving the real drug or the placebo. Some people who think that they are receiving the real drug but who are actually receiving the placebo will experience what is known as the *placebo effect*. In other words, they will experience some change or improvement – but, of course, this cannot be attributed to the drug!

In a *double-blind study*, the participants are allocated to the respective 'test' and 'placebo' groups by an independent researcher, who plays no part in collecting the data about the drug's effects. The researchers who collect and analyse the data do not know which of the participants are in the treatment group and which are receiving the placebo. When the data have been collected and fully analysed, the independent researcher will reveal to the other researchers which participants belong to which group. The aim of all of this is to minimise potential bias and clarify the 'cause and effect' relationship between dependent and independent variables.

Table 9.3 **Advantages and limitations of experiments**

Advantages	Limitations
● The reliability of data collected in experiments tends to be very high, as experiments can be duplicated in exactly the same circumstances ● 'Hard' quantitative data is produced, allowing statistical, analysis and comparison between changes in experimental circumstances ● The 'scientific' status of the experiment gives it a lot of prestige and credibility with potential participants	● The researcher can only collect data on a very specific and narrow topic – the relationship between two variables. There is no flexibility beyond this ● The validity of data can be suspect as the experimenter cannot be certain that he or she has under control all the non-experimental variables. Additionally, the validity may be questioned because what happens in the laboratory, under controlled conditions, may not happen in the less controlled real world ● The use of human beings in experimental situations raises many difficult ethical issues – people have feelings and rights that chemicals do not have!

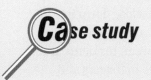

Case study

Example of research using an experimental strategy

Fader, M., Pettersson, L., Dean, G. *et al*. (1999) The selection of female urinals: results of a multicentre evaluation. *British Journal of Nursing*, **8**, 918–925.

This study tested 13 types of reusable female urinal that allow women to empty their bladders while in bed. Each urinal was evaluated by approximately 30 community-based women for a period of 1 week. The participants kept a diary of urinal usage and spills, and filled in a product evaluation form.

Reflective activity

Considering an experimental strategy

Check your progress so far by working through each of the following questions. Write down your responses to each prompt to demonstrate that you have thought through the various aspects involved in using an experimental strategy.

1. Give an example where an experiment would be the most suitable strategy for a research investigation

2. How is data collected when an experimental design is used?

3. What are your dependent and independent variables?

4. Can there be any ethical problems with experimental research?

Case studies

The case study strategy involves a systematic investigation into a single individual, event or situation: in other words, the researcher studies a single example, or case, of some phenomenon. The chosen case can be a person, group or situation that is researched because of its uniqueness and rarity value. Alternatively, the case might be chosen because it is a typical example of a type of person, group or situation.

Case study research is often conducted over a long period of time, so that detailed, in-depth data can be obtained. Case study researchers value depth more than breadth in their data. A common reason given for doing this is that case studies can 'illuminate the general by looking at the particular'.

Case study research is widely used in the social care, social science and health-care fields as it allows researchers to study in detail the relationships of individuals and small groups in their 'natural settings'. For example, when large mental hospitals began to close down in the 1980s, a number of case studies were conducted to find out how the closure process affected relationships between residents and staff. The research findings from these studies gave managers and staff a better insight into the closure process and its impact on various people involved.

Case study research is sometimes described as being 'holistic'. This is because researchers are keen to understand how the various elements and relationships within the case study setting work together. The researcher can then explain why certain things happen in the setting, rather than simply stating that they do.

Researchers who conduct case study research make use of a variety of data collection methods, including interviews, questionnaires, observations and analysis of documents. A case study researcher will adopt a 'horses for courses' approach to data collection and use whatever methods seem most appropriate in the situation. An advantage of this is that data can be validated by triangulation of methods (see Chapter 10).

In choosing a case study research design it is important to avoid disturbing the 'natural setting' that is being studied. Case study researchers place a great deal of value on not manipulating variables in the case study setting, as they wish to study events and relationships as they naturally occur.

Selecting a case to study

A case study strategy for a research project requires the researcher to choose one example of the class of thing that they wish to study. Then they need to justify their choice of case! How can this be done? Case study researchers have justified their decisions by saying that their chosen case is:

- A typical example of something, and therefore they have chosen it because this will allow them to generalise their findings to other similar cases
- An extreme example of something, and therefore they can study in depth the particularly unusual quality or factor that makes the case extreme.

As well as these justifications, many case study researchers explain their choice of case on pragmatic grounds. For example, a particular case may be chosen because it is more convenient or practical than some other possible case. This is acceptable as long as it is not the only or main reason for selecting a particular case to study.

The pros and cons of a case study strategy

Using a case study strategy has its advantages and drawbacks for small-scale project research. The decision to undertake a case study needs to be weighed up in the light of what is required, what the study is likely to achieve and what is felt about the other strategies open to the researcher.

Table 9.4 The case for and against the case study

For	Against
• A case study strategy is ideal for collecting data on subtle and complex social situations • You won't need to try to impose any control over events or variables, as you would if you used an experimental strategy • Case studies are generally manageable for people who wish to do small-scale project research, because their focus is limited to a defined setting, a group of people or even an individual	• The extent to which findings can be generalised beyond the case example that is studied is questionable – generalisations may not be possible or, if they are made, may not be credible • A case study will generally produce 'soft' qualitative data, which is acceptable if you are seeking a descriptive account but not so good if you are interested in also obtaining 'hard' factual data that will allow you to make statistical comparisons • You will have to negotiate access to the case study setting and ensure that you find ways of limiting the effect of your presence on the 'natural' behaviour and processes of the setting

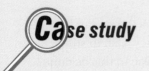

Case study

Example of research using a case study strategy

Atwal, A. (2002) Nurses' perception of discharge planning in acute health care: a case study in one British teaching hospital. *Journal of Advanced Nursing*, **39**, 450–458.

Nineteen nurses from one hospital were interviewed to identify their perceptions of the discharge process. Observations were also made of the multidisciplinary discharge planning communication. It found that aspects of discharge planning were sometimes ignored and that discharge planning was rarely co-ordinated because of lack of time.

Reflective activity

Considering a case study strategy

Check your progress so far by working through each of the following questions. Write down your responses to each prompt to demonstrate that you have thought through the various aspects involved in using a case study strategy.

1. When would a case study be the most suitable strategy for a research investigation?
2. How and why might a particular 'case' be selected?
3. What data collection methods can be used in a case study?
4. What can the researcher do to avoid disturbing the natural behaviour of the case study setting?
5. Can researchers generalise their findings beyond the case study setting?

Action research

Action research is a relatively new form of research strategy. It has gained a lot of popularity with health and social-care practitioners in particular. Action research has become strongly associated with small-scale, problem-solving research that has a practice development goal. In essence, action research is a strategy for investigating and solving problems, and a way of introducing and evaluating change. As a strategy, action research provides an opportunity to identify real problems and then to participate in and evaluate the effects of implementing possible solutions. Action research is really based on a cyclical process that could – in theory at least – never end.

Action research can be used within both a positivistic and a naturalistic approach to research. As with case study research, the action researcher can use many forms of data collection method.

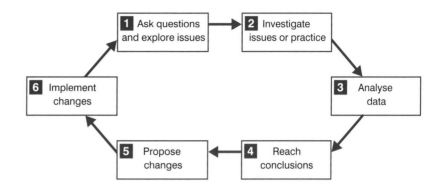

Figure 9.2 *The cyclical process of action research*

The approach and data collection methods used tend to depend on the disciplinary background of the researcher.

Action research is distinctive in that it encourages participatory research: in other words, action researchers encourage the 'researched' to participate in the research investigation as collaborators. In most research designs there is an assumption that the researcher is 'the expert', and that participants won't play an active part in conducting or providing feedback on the research process until it is completed. The participation encouraged by action research results in a shift in power, or 'democratisation', within the research process. This can be seen as positive and ethical, because it gives the 'researched'

Table 9.5 Advantages and limitations of action research

Advantages	Limitations
● An action research strategy allows the researcher to look at practical problems and feed into solutions and changes	● Action research is typically small-scale and local to an organisation – this limits the representativeness and the generalisability of any findings
● It enables the researcher to develop his or her own practice	● 'Variables' cannot be manipulated, as the research is conducted into ongoing activities and processes
● It can provide benefits to participants and organisations	● Action research is ethically constrained: it usually affects people's lives so the researcher must be in a position to take responsibility for all consequences and limit any risks to those affected
● There is democratisation of the process through participation by the 'researched'	● Within the partnership framework of action research, the ownership and leadership of the research process and findings can be contested
	● The researcher needs to be a practitioner in some sense
	● Action researchers are not detached or impartial – therefore it does not fit with a 'positivistic' scientific approach

an important role and 'voice' in the research process. On the other hand, it can lead to problems if leadership of the research process becomes blurred.

In considering the possibility of using this strategy, the researcher needs to bear in mind that action research has to be undertaken as part of some form of practice. To be able to identify and implement 'change' through your research, an action researcher needs to have some kind of 'practitioner' role. It is unlikely that full-time students would have such a role outside of their college/university life.

Case study

Example of research using an action research approach

Davis, S. and Marsden, R. (2001) Disabled people in hospital: evaluating the Clinical Nurse Specialist role. *Nursing Standard*, **15**, 33–37.

This research evaluated a newly established CNS in disability role in a large acute hospital. It used data from a questionnaire given to 38 clients (response rate 24), general discussion and feedback from patients and other carers, admission records and diary reflections made by the CNS. The CNS was able to identify problems such as a lack of awareness of disability in clinical staff, and acted on these findings implementing teaching sessions for staff.

Reflective activity

Considering an action research strategy

Check your progress so far by working through each of the following questions. Write down your responses to each prompt to demonstrate that you have thought through the various aspects involved in carrying out action research.

1. Give an example of when action research would be the most suitable strategy for a research investigation.
2. Why do action researchers need to have a work role in which they are 'practitioners' in some way?
3. Can you think of something that you would like to change through action research activity?
4. To what extent is it possible to generalise the findings from an action research setting?

*RRRRR***Rapid recap**

Check your progress so far by working through each of the following questions.

1. Why is random sampling a useful method for choosing a research group from a large population?
2. What is the role of a 'control group' in an experimental study?
3. Could an in-depth single interview with a patient be described as a case study?

If you have difficulty with more than one of the questions, read through the section again to refresh your understanding before moving on.

Further reading

Abrams, K. and Scragg, A. (1996) Quantitative methods in nursing research. *Journal of Advanced Nursing*, **23**, 1008–1015.

Altman, D. and Bland, J. (1999) How to randomise. *British Medical Journal*, **319**, 703–704.

Hillier, V. and Gibbs, A. (1996) Calculations to determine sample size. *Nurse Researcher*, **3**, 27–34.

Wood, N. (2001) Different questions, different designs, in: *The Health Project Book: A handbook for new researchers in the field of health*. Routledge, London, pp. 13–27.

Research designs

The initial planning stages of a research investigation include:

- Deciding on a research topic
- Gathering background information
- Narrowing the topic down to a specific aspect or research problem
- Producing a research question, and perhaps an hypothesis
- Choosing a research strategy

However, there are still a few more planning activities to do before you can launch into data collection. One of these is to choose a research design. The main purpose of a research design is to plan and explain how you will find answers to your research question(s) and how you will put your research strategy into action. At this stage in the research process it is important to ensure that a valid, workable and manageable solution is chosen for the particular research project and that appropriate resources are available.

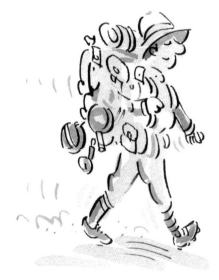

Good planning and preparation always pays off when the research is under way

Types of research design

There are a number of different ways of defining research designs. Figure 10.1 divides these into categories according to:

- The number of contacts made with respondents
- The reference period, or 'time-frame', of the investigation.

This will identify the number of data collection contacts.

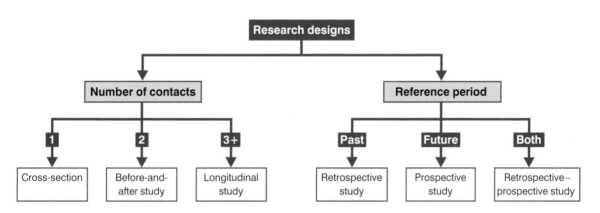

Figure 10.1 *Types of research design*

Cross-sectional study design

Collection of data on a single occasion can be described as a cross-sectional study. It will give a snapshot, or cross-section, 'picture' of the phenomenon and the people who are being studied, at a particular moment in time.

Cross-sectional studies are the simplest research study designs and are ideal for a student research project (depending on the research question). An important point to remember is that cross-sectional designs result in a 'still' picture. They cannot be used to measure any kind of change.

Before-and-after designs

Many researchers want to measure the extent to which change has occurred in some phenomenon and they need to select a before-and-after study design. This is also called a pre-test/post-test design and is often (but not always) used by researchers who are conducting experiments or evaluating the impact of a change in practices or policies. This type of design is really two cross-sectional studies conducted on the same population at different moments in time. Change is measured by comparing the two sets of findings.

By its very nature of involving data from two moments in time, this form of research design probably leads to more data collection and analysis work than in a single-contact cross-sectional study. This also means that more resources are required, and so a before-and-after study is often financially more expensive to conduct. There are a number of other limitations or weaknesses inherent in before-and-after research designs. These do not always occur but may do depending on the nature of the study.

- The **extraneous variable** problem means, basically, that researchers cannot be sure that the change they are seeking to measure is all caused by the factors being studied. 'Extraneous variables' are factors or influences that are outside researcher control, and are often things that may not even have been considered. The problem is that there will be no overall way of quantifying the extent of change caused by extraneous variables.

- The **maturation effect** problem refers to the fact that the respondents may well, especially if they are children or adolescents, change as a result of maturation between the 'before' and 'after' data collection times.

- The **reactive effect** problem refers to the situation in which the data collection method (such as a questionnaire or a series of interview questions) actually educates the respondents. This will, in itself, result in some change in their attitudes or behaviour towards the topic being studied.

Most before-and-after study designs have extraneous variable and reactive effect problems. If this type of research design is chosen, researchers should think through the ways in which these problems may impact on their findings. The findings won't necessarily be invalidated but the potential ways in which these problems may have impacted on the study do need to be acknowledged.

More fundamentally, careful decision-making is required to assess whether sufficient time is available to use a before-and-after design.

Longitudinal study design

A longitudinal study design is used to study a pattern of change over time, or when factual information is required on a continuing basis. Studies of patterns of disease and death rates use longitudinal study designs.

As you have probably worked out, this design involves repeated data collection contacts with respondents. These contacts usually take place over a relatively long period. This feature of the design makes a longitudinal study an unlikely choice for a student research project.

Despite this, the period of time between data collection contacts is not fixed and the intervals do not have to be of the same length. For example, in an unorthodox longitudinal study, data could be collected every other day, or two or three times a week. In practice, longitudinal studies usually involve repeated data collection episodes over periods of months or years, not days.

In essence, longitudinal studies are cross-sectional studies repeated a number of times. They are an extension of the before-and-after type of design and, as such, may involve the same weaknesses or limitations. An additional problem of longitudinal study designs is the *conditioning effect*. This occurs where respondents learn what is expected of them and then either lose interest or behave in the way they think the researcher wants them to. In effect, they have been 'conditioned' by repeated experiences to respond to questions in particular ways, and end up giving their responses without putting any real thought into them.

The reference period

A second factor that affects the research design is the reference period, or time-frame, for the study. Again, there are three possibilities – retrospective, prospective and retrospective and prospective.

Retrospective study design

This type of study investigates the past. It either involves looking at data that has already been collected for the period concerned or is based on what respondents can remember about the situation or problem.

Prospective study design

This type of study design investigates the likely future prevalence of a phenomenon. Researchers using this design consider what the outcome of a situation or event might be.

Retrospective–prospective study design

This type of study design is a hybrid of the previous two. The researcher looks at past trends or data on a phenomenon and then studies what might happen in the future. Before-and-after studies are likely to be retrospective–prospective designs. Part of the data will have been collected before the intervention that is being studied, and then the respondents are studied to find out what effect the intervention has had.

Table 10.1 **The advantages and limitations of research designs**

Number of data collection contacts	Type of design	Advantages	Limitations
One only	Cross-sectional study	• Simple to plan • Cheap to do • Easy to analyse	• Gives a snapshot only • Cannot measure change
Two	Before-and-after study	• Measures change or impact of interventions between two moments in time	• More work than a cross-sectional study • Can be expensive and time-consuming • Respondents can change between before and after points; data then lacks validity • You cannot be sure of the effect of extraneous variables on findings
Three or more	Longtitudinal study	• Can measure the pattern of change over time	• Involves extensive data collection and analysis • Requires more resources than cross-sectional or before-and-after studies • You need to have a relatively long period of time available to collect data • Data can be affected by the conditioning effect

Reflective activity

Considering research designs

Check your progress so far by working through each of the following questions. Write down your responses to each prompt to demonstrate that you have thought through the various aspects involved in using different research designs.

1. What are the two factors which need to be considered in choosing a research design?
2. What is meant by the terms 'conditioning effect' and 'maturation effect' in research designs?
3. How can you minimise the problems that might occur with multicontact approaches from a research design perspective?

Selecting data collection methods

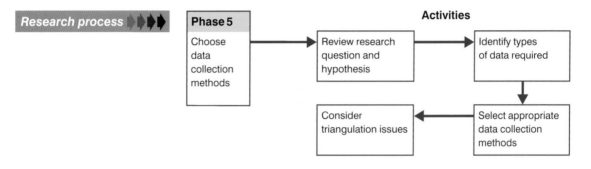

Figure 10.2 *Phase 5: Choosing data collection methods*

In the next section we will look at what many people associate with 'doing research' – getting the data. The focus here will be on the main options for obtaining primary data. It is important, as a researcher, to be open-minded and creative in the selection of methods and to weigh up the strengths and weaknesses of different data collection methods while bearing in mind your research question(s), the design and the resources you have available. Following an examination of each data collection method an example is given to illustrate how this has been used in a completed research study. What will quickly become clear as you look at 'real life' examples is that different data collection methods are often used together within one study.

Questionnaires

Questionnaires are simply lists of pre-written questions and sometimes also include scales. Researchers typically include a variety of *closed questions, rating scales, semantic differential items* and *'forced choice' items* in questionnaires. Explanations and examples of each of these terms can be found in Table 10.2.

These three kinds of questionnaire 'response item' allow researchers to collect large amounts of quantitative data that can be analysed statistically. Researchers who are adopting a positivist approach often make use of questionnaires to survey a representative sample of the population in whom they are interested.

Table 10.2 **Explanations and examples of items used in questionnaires**	
Explanation	**Example**
Closed questions offer limited scope for response. They are usually of the 'yes/no' variety or can offer three or more choices	Do you smoke cigarettes? Which of these shifts do you prefer working – early, late or night?
A **semantic differential** scale asks the respondent to choose a point between two different 'poles'/words that most represents the intensity of their view or feelings	I find the thought of working in the Accident and Emergency Department Scary ————————————————— Exciting
Rating scales (Likert scale) require the respondent to indicate a degree of preference or agreement from a limited range of choices	Choose the item nearest to your own view on the statement: 'Student occupational therapists learn a lot from undertaking specialist clinical placements' ● Strongly agree ● Agree ● Neither agree or disagree ● Disagree ● Strongly disagree
'Forced choice' items set out a possible range of responses, from which respondents then choose. They are generally used to obtain factual/numeric information	Which of the following age groups do you currently belong to? ● 18–19 ● 23–24 ● 20–21 ● 25 and over ● 22–23

Researchers who adopt a naturalistic approach use questionnaire methods much less frequently. Where they are used in naturalistic research, questionnaires are likely to be less structured and less restrictive in terms of the responses that they permit, or are used for triangulation purposes (see page 104). Typically, the naturalistic researcher would include more open questions. These allow for a variety of individual responses and fit better with the aim of getting an 'insider view' of a situation. Open questions also help researchers to avoid accidentally introducing any of their preconceptions, and protect the validity of the data.

Table 10.3 **The advantages and limitations of questionnaires as a data collection method**	
Advantages	**Limitations**
• They can be a cheap and efficient way of collecting data • They can collect a large amount of data relatively quickly • They are relatively reliable as a method of data collection • A comparison of respondent's answers is possible	• They can be difficult to get people to complete • The response rate of postal questionnaires is particularly low • Respondents often have a limited choice of answers. They may not reveal or express their real views or attitudes if they do not match the 'forced choices'. Data collection possibilities are pre-limited by the researcher, as respondents can only provide responses to a restricted range of questions or scales • Unless the questionnaire is conducted face-to-face, the researcher cannot be sure of the true identity of the respondent • The respondents tend to be people who have stronger views or attitudes on the subject being surveyed • If the questionnaire is posted, the researcher cannot be sure that respondents have understood the questions and cannot use follow-up questions to explore unusual answers

Reflective activity

Considering questionnaires

Check your progress so far by working through each of the following questions. Write down your responses to each prompt to demonstrate that you have thought through the various aspects involved in using questionnaires.

1. Why is a questionnaire a good way of getting data for an investigation?
2. What are the advantages and disadvantages of administering a questionnaire face-to-face in comparison to by post?
3. How can the confidentiality of respondents be protected when a questionnaire is used?
4. What would be an acceptable amount of time to expect a respondent to take to answer a questionnaire?

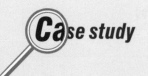

Case study

An example of a research study that used questionnaires

Timmins, F. and Kaliszer, M. (2002) Absenteeism among nursing students – fact or fiction? *Journal of Nursing Management*, **10**, 251–256.

In this retrospective study involving third-year students at two hospital sites, the attendance records of students were analysed. In addition, a questionnaire was given to student nurses asking them to identify the reasons why they were absent.

The findings indicated that a total of 4% of the days of the course were lost through absenteeism, that mostly this involved periods of 3 days or less, and that 73% of 1-day absences occurred on Mondays and Fridays. These absences occurred more frequently from lectures than from clinical placements and the students identified personal, social commitments and stress as the main reasons for absenteeism.

The Delphi method

The Delphi method involves systematically collecting information and judgements from a range of experts on a particular issue or subject (Jones and Hunter 2000). Questions covering the issue investigated are sent, often in the form of a questionnaire, to the expert panel members, who complete these individually and return them to the researcher. The researcher identifies the level of consensus among the experts' responses. The combined and analysed responses are then sent back to the expert panel members with their original response to the questions for them to further rate or rank. This allows them to reconsider their original views and responses. This re-examination of their responses can be done many times. A final consensus on the issue is then reached.

Table 10.4 **The advantages and limitations of the Delphi method of data collection**

Advantages	Limitations
• Participants have time to consider their answers and do not have direct contact with the researcher, who might influence their opinions	• Participants may not have the time to respond on more than one occasion to a request for data
• Takes less time and effort than individual interviews, and is an economical way of getting attitudinal data from a number of experts in a particular field	• There is little guidance as to the size of the expert panel needed and the number of rounds before consensus is achieved
• Participants can revise, add to and retract their views during various rounds of data collection	• May be difficult to determine 'experts' on a particular issue

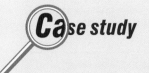

Case study

An example of a research study that used the Delphi method

Roberts-Davis, M. and Read, S. (2001) Clinical role clarification: using the Delphi method to establish similarities and differences between nurse practitioners and clinical nurse specialists. *Journal of Clinical Nursing*, **10**, 33–43.

This study used the Delphi technique by contacting nurses, educators, purchasers, providers and representatives of professional bodies and tried to achieve consensus about the parameters and competencies of nurse practitioners and clinical nurse specialists.

Interviews

Interviews are similar to questionnaires in that they are organised around a series of questions and rely on an interviewee being able to answer and tell the 'truth' as they see it. However, interviews are more than long-winded alternatives to questionnaires.

Interviews can be used within either a positivist or a naturalistic research approach, depending on the extent to which they are pre-structured by the researcher. People who adopt a positivist approach will tend to produce a more highly structured schedule of questions that they ask all interviewees. Sometimes researchers who use these *structured interviews* will read out the questions and a limited choice of possible answers to the respondents.

Researchers who adopt a naturalistic approach tend to use *semi-structured* or *unstructured interviews*. In these situations, the researcher has fewer predetermined questions and is more likely to let the interview develop as a 'guided conversation', according to the interests and wishes of the interviewee. The fact that the researcher is physically present during data-gathering can be both an advantage (people may be more likely to answer questions fully, and the interviewer can ask for further explanation and give clarification) and a disadvantage (their presence may have a 'biasing' effect on responses) of interviews over questionnaires. The advantages and disadvantages of semi-structured interviews are outlined in more detail in Table 10.5.

Table 10.5 **The advantages and limitations of interviews as a data collection method**	
Advantages	**Limitations**
• It is possible to avoid too much pre-judgement if the questions are not predetermined; the researcher can obtain the interviewee's 'real' views and beliefs	• The validity of data is always suspect – it is never possible to be 100% sure either that interviewees are not deliberately lying or that they can recall the 'truth' correctly
• Semi-structured interviews give the researcher an opportunity to 'probe' what the respondent says; the researcher can also discover and make use of unexpected and unforeseen information as it is revealed	• Recording information can be difficult. Writing down what people say is difficult and can be intrusive. It is hard to keep up and it interrupts the flow of an interview if you keep stopping to write. Tape recording the interview is much better but introduces confidentiality issues and may cause respondents to limit what they say
• The depth of information is improved, because the interviewer can explore what the respondent 'really means' or 'really believes', as s/he talks more freely	• People usually give too much information in semi- and unstructured interviews; most of what they say is not usable and goes into the subject in too much depth
• Response rates can be very good, as the interviewer is present to ensure completion of data collection	• Interviews take a long time to complete, and even longer to transcribe into a written record of what was said
• The researcher can give help and guidance, explaining questions and giving additional information where it is needed	• The reliability of 'data' is poor – it is very difficult to compare responses between respondents, because they may not have been asked exactly the same questions and, as a result, can produce very different data

Reflective activity

Considering interviews

Check your progress so far by working through each of the following questions. Write down your responses to each prompt to demonstrate that you have thought through the various aspects involved in using interviews to collect data.

1. How does the level of structure within an interview affect data collection?
2. What factors would need to be taken into account regarding where interviews are to be carried out?
3. What would you consider to be the right length of time for an interview?
4. What methods can be used to record what respondents say and what are the advantages and disadvantages of each?

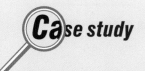

Case study

Examples of research studies that used interviews

Costello, J. (2002) Do not resuscitate orders and older patients: findings from an ethnographic study of hospital wards for older people. *Journal of Advanced Nursing*, **39**, 491–499.

In this qualitative study, semi-structured interviews and participant observation of nurses and doctors looking after terminally ill older patients found that 'Do Not Resuscitate' orders were socially constructed.

Vrij, A., Edward, K. and Bull, R. (2001) People's insight into their own behaviour and speech content while lying. *British Journal of Psychology*, **92**, 373–389.

Student nurses were given a film to watch and were then interviewed twice about the film they had just seen. One interview involved them telling the truth, and the other requested that they lie about the film. All the interviews were videotaped and transcribed. Participants were asked to indicate on a questionnaire whether they thought they had shown stereotypical behaviours and speech when lying. The findings indicated that the student nurses believed the content of their speech was less stereotypical of lying than their behaviours and this was found to be opposite to the comparative observational data.

Focus groups

Focus groups have become increasingly popular as a method of collecting data, particularly in qualitative studies. This method has a long history of use in market research. It has a lot in common with the interview method but, unlike interviews, which are usually held one-to one,

Table 10.6 The advantages and limitations of focus groups as a data collection method

Advantages	Limitations
● Provides an opportunity for in-depth discussion and to examine the attitudes and group dynamics affecting a particular issue	● Requires a skilled researcher who can moderate the discussions in the group and collect data concurrently
● Takes less time and effort than individual interviews and is an economical way of obtaining the views of a number of people	● Can produce results that are peculiar to the particular mix of people and their group dynamics – for example, one very vocal participant can affect the whole group
● Useful in understanding different perspectives where there may be a communication gap (e.g. between managers, health-care professionals and patients/service users)	● It is not usually possible to generalise from a focus group study as they tend to be small-scale and limited
● People are more aware of their own perspective when confronted with active disagreement, and they analyse their views more intensely than in a one-to-one interview	● Requires eight to 12 participants and non-attendance can affect the working of the focus group

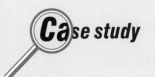

Examples of research studies that used focus groups

McHugh, G. and Thomas, G. (2001) Patient satisfaction with chronic pain management. *Nursing Standard*, **15**, 33–38.
Focus groups were used to investigate the patients' experience of chronic pain.
Evans, K. (2001) Expectations of newly qualified nurses. *Nursing Standard*, **15**, 33–38.
Nine newly qualified nurses were asked in a focus group to discuss their concerns and expectations during their role transition from student to staff nurse.

focus groups get together eight to 12 people in a discussion-based interview to generate data. The group is focused and staged by a member of the research team acting as moderator (Morrison and Peoples 1999).

Participant observation

In a participant observation study, researchers enter the group or situation that they are studying. Participant observers try to 'get to know' the group or situation 'from the inside'. They need to try to understand the motives and meanings of the people whom they are studying, from the point of view of those people. The aim of this is for the researcher to gain a deeper insight into the real way of life, beliefs and activities of the group in their 'natural setting'. It is believed that the researcher's own experience of the group will give them access to data that might not be elicited (drawn out) by a questionnaire or interview.

In both interviewing and observational research situations, people may more obviously react to the presence of the researcher when they know research is taking place. This is termed the *Hawthorne effect*. This expression originates from a study in 1939 by Roethlisberger and Dickinson, who were studying the activity of the workers in the Western Electric Works Hawthorne plant in Chicago. The researchers noted that workers' productivity increased when the working environment was improved by better lighting conditions. However, they also found that, when the lighting conditions were made worse, worker productivity still improved. The conclusion they reached was that the workers were responding to the presence of the researchers and the realisation that they were participants in a research study. As a researcher you should be aware of the possibility that you may have an influence on the findings.

Participant observation is closely associated with the naturalistic approach to research. It is a data collection method that most positivistic researchers reject because the 'participant' researcher does not remain detached or 'separate' from the research participants or the situation. Because of the danger that participant observation may not produce objective data, researchers often use other methods, such as interviews, alongside it to provide complementary data.

Observational methods can be *overt* – where the researcher identifies him/herself and their purpose to the people being studied – or *covert* – where the researcher's identity and purpose remain secret. The advantages and limitations of participant observation as a data collection method are outlined in Table 10.7.

Table 10.7 **The advantages and limitations of participant observation**

Advantages	Limitations
• Observations of 'real' life in natural settings give access to highly valid data	• Researchers may not be able to retain their objectivity or avoid becoming involved in the life of the group. This is sometimes referred to as 'going native'. Researchers may also influence behaviour or events in the research setting if they become too involved
• Observation can produce data that is rich in meaning and may give access to otherwise 'hidden' data	
• Participant observers can often obtain detailed data over a long period of time	• Participant observers may never really understand the group or setting if they are unable to appreciate the deep meaning and significance of behaviour from the standpoint of a detached outsider
• Covert participant observation may be the only way of accessing 'hidden' data or hostile groups	• Participant observation studies tend to be small scale and the group being studied may also not be representative of any other social group (therefore findings cannot be generalised)
• Researchers do not have to decide what they are looking for in advance of beginning their study – they can make decisions about what is and is not significant behaviour as events occur and unfold naturally	• Covert observation has serious ethical implications and problems associated with it – for example, informed consent is not obtained when covert observation is carried out
	• The reliability of observational data collection methods is relatively low, because observations are often personal and non-repeatable

Non-participant observation is less commonly used within research studies. Where it is, the researcher observes a situation or a group of people from a distance and as an 'outsider'. This might occur, for example, where a researcher wishes to use an observational tool to record actions or behaviours as they occur or to analyse a video of a particular setting.

The level of participation that researchers choose tends to depend on their research skills and experience and also the approach that they are taking to the research investigation. For example, positivistic researchers are more likely to use non-participant observation whereas naturalistic researchers have a tendency towards greater participant observation.

Reflective activity

Considering observational methods

Check your progress so far by working through each of the following questions. Write down your responses to each prompt to demonstrate that you have thought through the various aspects involved in using participant observation methods.

1. If you wished to study your own student group how would you gain access to the group to observe?
2. What can be done to avoid disturbing the natural behaviour of the group?
3. Would it be acceptable to undertake covert research in a health-care setting?
4. How can observations be recorded?

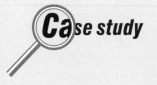

Case study

An example of a research study that used participant observation

Holyoake, D. (2002) Male identity in mental health nursing. *Nursing Standard*, **16**, 33–37.

This study involved participant observation of male nurses working in mental health setting. This was combined with in-depth interviews. The researcher identified the notion of 'soft masculinity' that involved the need for male nurses to demonstrate gentleness and caring, balanced with maintaining a sense of their masculine identity.

Theory and **Practice**

A recent addition to health care research designs is the study of narratives. An example of this could be a patient's verbal account of their own illness story. Narratives have:

- A finite time sequence (including a beginning, a series of events, and an ending)
- A narrator and a listener
- A concern with events, but also with feelings and motives
- The opportunity for the narrator to choose what to tell and what to omit
- Interesting content for the listener that invites interpretation

Documentary analysis

The analysis of documents is a data collection technique that is associated with historians and other humanities researchers. In the same way as historians, health and social-care professionals who use documentary analysis techniques need to establish the validity and authenticity of any documents they are going to analyse.

One type of document that can be analysed is the diary. As a health-care student you may be expected to keep a 'reflective diary' during your training. This could be systematically analysed within a research study about student learning and the role of reflective diaries. Patients may also be asked to keep a diary of their symptoms and health problems. Again, these can (with consent) be analysed to give a qualitative account of the introduction of a new treatment.

The term 'document' does suggest that the data is in a textual format , and often this is the case. However, documentary analysis can also be applied to spoken narratives and visual information, such as art. There are a wide range of potential documentary data sources, including archives, textbooks, academic journals, curricula, official reports, minutes of meetings, medical case notes, letters, television programmes and autobiographies. This list shows that sources can be 'public' (produced in a situation that is open to public scrutiny) or 'private' (directed at a restricted audience and likely to be more detailed and frank).

Table 10.8 The advantages and limitations of documentary sources of data

Advantages	Limitations
● Provides an opportunity for rich data with easier access	● The social context in which the document was created and the purpose of the document may be unclear
● Can provide access to large quantities of data in a cost-effective time period	● The passage of time since their creation may make documents difficult to interpret
● The date when the data has been produced is clear	● Deliberate distortion or misrepresentation within the document can have occurred

---

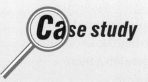

Case study

An example of a research study that used documentary analysis

Scholes, J., Endacott, R. and Chellel, A. (2000) A formula for diversity: a review of critical care curricula. *Journal of Clinical Nursing*, **9**, 382–390

Curriculum documents for critical care courses run by different educational institutions were analysed. This was combined with telephone survey data from lecturers and clinical managers. The study found a great diversity in critical care courses.

Triangulation – covering all bases

Professional and academic researchers tend to use 'triangulation' techniques in their research investigations. Triangulation is a kind of 'belt and braces' or insurance policy approach that is used to try to counter the weaknesses that exist in different methods of data collection and analysis. In essence, when researchers triangulate, they use more than one method of data collection and analysis.

In the end I decided on three main lines of approach: in-depth interviews, participant observation and a questionnaire. From the interview I hoped to understand the individual as an individual. From the participant observation I hoped to observe the interpersonal level (relationships between members) and from the questionnaire I hoped to see patterns and relationships about which I could only generalise from a large number of respondents.

Barker 1984

The use of multiple methods of data collection and analysis allows a researcher to benefit from the advantages of each method used while trying to minimise the impact of their individual weaknesses. For example, a researcher might decide to use an unstructured interview at the beginning of the study, to identify what the key issues and terms were, and then use this information to develop a more structured set of interview questions, or a questionnaire.

Triangulation-by-method and triangulation-by-analysis enable a researcher to explore various aspects of the same topic, looking at it from different sides or angles. In terms that we have used previously, researchers can collect both quantitative and qualitative data from primary and secondary sources. Research investigations that use triangulation tend to be based on one main data collection method that is supplemented by others.

When researchers plan their projects they need to consider how data is to be obtained, what the strengths and weaknesses of the chosen data collection methods are and whether triangulation by method is necessary. If a data collection method has validity weaknesses (e.g. interviews) it may be triangulated with another method in which validity is strong (e.g. participant observation). Similarly, if the method has reliability weaknesses (e.g. participant observation) it could be combined with another in which reliability is strong (e.g. questionnaires).

RRRRRRapid recap

Check your progress so far by working through each of the following questions.

1. What is the difference between a cross-sectional study design and a before-and-after research design?

2. If you were researching the need for dietary supplements for elderly patients while hospitalised, what would be the advantages and disadvantages of the following data collection methods?
   - Questionnaire
   - Delphi Method
   - Interview
   - Focus group
   - Participant observation
   - Documentary analysis

3. What is meant by the term 'triangulation' in relation to research design?

If you have difficulty with more than one of the questions, read through the section again to refresh your understanding before moving on.

References

Barker, E. (1984) *The Making of a Moonie*. Blackwell, Oxford.

Jones, J. and Hunter, D. (2000) Using the Delphi and nominal group technique in health services research, in: *Qualitative Research in Health Care*, 2nd edn (eds C. Pope and N. Mays). British Medical Journal, London, pp. 40–49.

Morrison, R. and Peoples, L. (1999) Using focus group methodology in nursing. *Journal of Continuing Education in Nursing*, **30**, 62–65.

Roethlisberger, F. and Dickinson, W. (1939) *Management and the Worker*. Harvard University Press, Cambridge, MA.

Further reading

Clancy, M. (2002) Overview of research designs. *Emergency Medicine Journal*, **19**, 546–549.

Foss, C. (2002) The value of combining qualitative and quantitative approaches in nursing research by means of a method triangulation. *Journal of Advanced Nursing*, **40**, 242–248.

Wood, N. (2001) *The health project book: a handbook for new researchers in the field of health*. Routledge, London.

11 Ethical considerations and developing a research proposal

Research investigations are associated with 'progress', 'discovery' and 'improvement' in our understanding of the world. They are generally seen as a good thing. However, in order to be acceptable, any research investigation must be *ethical*. The *ethics* of research are concerned with the standards of behaviour and the practical procedures that researchers are expected to follow. Questions about what is *moral* (right as opposed to wrong) are indeed a part of research ethics. However, researchers do not usually have to become involved in deep philosophical thinking about the big moral issues that are a general feature of research.

Thinking about ethics

Most research involving human subjects has ethical implications. On one hand these may be very minor and the research will, in most cases, cause no harm. However, in extreme cases the implications of research can be long-lasting and detrimental. Researchers need to find ways of applying a limited set of *ethical principles* to their research investigation.

Ethical research in health care is important because it often involves patients, staff and students. Your concern with ethics should be driven by a genuine desire to protect the interests of participants rather than by any other concern you have about satisfying the needs of an Ethics Committee.

The key criteria that must be met before research is considered 'ethically acceptable' are as follows:

- **Protection of rights**: the participants' right to privacy and confidentiality should be protected
- **Protection from harm**: no harm should be done to others as a result of the research

- **Positive contribution**: some good or benefit should come out of the research investigation; it should result in a positive contribution to knowledge and human understanding
- **Honesty and integrity**: researchers should act in an honest way and be truthful and open in their methods and behaviour.

All research participants have a basic right to privacy and to be fully informed about what participation in a research investigation involves. Clear, practical ways of gaining informed consent and of protecting the confidentiality of the data obtained from participants are required to ensure that participants' rights are preserved.

Obtaining informed consent

Researchers must be able to demonstrate that their research participants have freely consented to being involved in the research investigation and that they have a full understanding of what the research involves. They must be aware of the aims of the research and of any risks that they may face if they participate. They must also be fully aware of what they will be required to do or will experience during the research investigation.

How is informed consent obtained?

Firstly, a short statement that explains the study and what is involved should be given to participants. This can be either read, shown or preferably given to each of the potential participants when the researcher or the researcher's assistants try to recruit them as a volunteer. When constructing an information sheet try to:

- Keep sentences short
- Avoid jargon or medical terms (explain them if they have to be used)
- Use subheadings and avoid long paragraphs
- Use a large enough font size (12pt or larger)
- Check it out on lay people to make sure that it is easy to read and understand.

It is an established principle that researchers should not trick people into unwittingly participating in research. A researcher must never lie to conceal the fact that they are doing research, and all participants in a research study should be willing volunteers.

Obtaining informed consent can sometimes be problematic. For example, informed consent is difficult to obtain from children and from people with learning disabilities. It is important to remember that some potential recruits are unable to fully understand the nature, requirements and risks involved in a research investigation. It would, therefore, be wrong to unwittingly involve such people in a research study if there were any doubts about their ability to give informed consent. It is also important that no inducements are used to encourage vulnerable people to be involved in a study. It is, however, acceptable to offer travelling expenses if a patient is expected to make additional visits to the outpatient department because of the monitoring required for a study they are participating in.

You may have read about research studies where the researcher deliberately carried out secret or 'covert' research. These studies usually involve an investigation into a subject that is very sensitive or that involves 'hidden' data. As such, the only way of gaining access to the 'data' was to carry out the study without informing the people being studied. In most circumstances, this is unethical. **You should not carry out a covert study for a student research project**.

A written consent form, which will require a signature from the participant and the researcher, should include the following information:

- That the participant is a volunteer and willing to take part in the study
- That the nature and purpose of, and any risks inherent in, the study have been explained to the participant
- The likely involvement, in terms of time, of the participant
- That the participant has had the opportunity to question the researcher
- That the participant is free to withdraw from the study at any time without needing to justify their decision.

An example of a consent form is included here to show how this information can be incorporated.

As well as gaining the consent of participants who will be involved in the study, the researcher will also need to gain the agreement of the manager in charge of the clinical area if data collection is to occur in a work setting. Written permission, often in the form of a supportive letter, will be required before data collection can go ahead.

CONSENT TO PARTICIPATE IN A RESEARCH STUDY

Student nurses' perceptions of what mentorship behaviours are helpful

Principal investigator: Steven Davis

- I am undertaking this small-scale research study as part of my studies to gain a BSc (Hons) Nursing Studies at the University of Health. Thank you for agreeing to take part in this research study. Your selection to participate in this study involved the use of a random selection process, and your participation is entirely voluntary.

- This study looks at the experiences of student nurses on clinical placements in hospital wards. The research aims to gain an in-depth insight into student nurses' perceptions of what mentorship behaviours are helpful.

- Your help with this study is entirely voluntary, and should you decide not to take part you will not be affected in any way. You may withdraw your consent at any time by notifying Steven Davis without prejudicing yourself. You will be interviewed once, for no longer than 40 minutes, at a time that is convenient to you. This interview will be tape-recorded and a copy of the typed transcripts from your interview will be sent to you. You may keep this copy of your data, and will be asked to check it for factual accuracy and to sanction its use within the study. You can also make any further comments and clarify issues at any time.

- Completion of the study is not expected before September 2005. No reports will contain your name, work location or any personal identifiers. Your participation will remain in absolute confidence.

- This is not a clinical study, and there is no payment involved, so thank you again for supporting this study.

- By signing this form you acknowledge that information has been provided about the research and your rights as a subject, and all questions have been answered to your satisfaction. If at any time you have any questions, Steven Davis can be contacted at [Telephone Number]. Dr David Stevens (University of Health) is the research supervisor. In signing this document you consent to being a participant in this research study.

Signed: _____

Interviewee _____ Date _____

Address data to be sent to _____

_____

_____

Interviewer _____ Date _____

Address for further information or questions. _____

_____

_____

Figure 11.1 *Example of a consent form*

Fulfilling ethical principles

Confidentiality

All research participants have a right to privacy. This includes the right to withdraw from the research investigation at any point if they wish to, the right to refuse to answer any question asked, and the right to remain anonymous and to have the confidentiality of their data protected. Information that personally identifies an individual or group of people must not be entered on to a computer without application and registration with the Data Protection Registrar. As this would normally be impractical for student projects, but is legally required by the Data Protection Act (1984), it is safer for students not to record any identifying information. Any confidential information should be destroyed at the end of the research study.

In research situations, confidentiality is taken to mean that the information, or data, given by a participant is not revealed to others who are not part of the research team, except in an anonymous form when the findings of the study are reported. It also means that the data obtained in the research study should only be used for the purposes of the research study. No part of it should be sold to, or be re-used by, people for other research or non-research purposes unless the participants have agreed to this. With a small-scale research study, researchers have to think carefully about how they can protect the confidentiality of participants. Merely changing participants' names can be ineffective as a way of protecting confidentiality in such circumstances.

Protection from harm

The golden rule of research is that the researcher should never do any harm to research participants or those who may be affected by the research. Professional researchers in health and social care need to clearly identify and document any, and all, of the risks that participants may face. Research that involved injuring, maiming or harming another person could never be ethically justifiable. Where a research study may have a negative impact on the physical or mental health of a participant, even to the extent of temporarily upsetting them, they should be fully informed of this risk, and the researcher should take every possible step to minimise any harm coming to them. **You should not, of course, engage in any research that may put your participants at physical or psychological risk in any way.**

Positive contribution

Ideally, a research study should do some good, or at least be of benefit to participants. Research should not be carried out for the sake of it, or simply to benefit the career or reputation of the researcher. As a student researcher you won't be expected to make a significant contribution to human knowledge and understanding through your study. It is appreciated that students may have to conduct research in order to qualify. However, you should still undertake your research with the aim of advancing your knowledge and understanding, and should avoid any kind of frivolous reason.

There are many situations in which research findings are not as expected, or where they are less than earth-shatteringly important. However, if research begins with a serious and legitimate intention and could potentially have a beneficial outcome – adding new knowledge to human understanding – it could be said to be ethically justifiable. It is not ethical if it is frivolous, involves illegal behaviour or unjustifiable suffering, or has no beneficial intention or purpose.

Honesty and integrity

The final ethical principle is linked to the above point, in that it is concerned with the standard of behaviour and integrity of researchers. There is a general expectation that researchers will be truthful and act with integrity. Data must be gathered carefully, findings reported honestly and any problems, errors or distortions acknowledged. Researchers must never falsify their data or make false claims that are not backed up by the data that they have. Sadly, researchers do not always live up to the 'ethical' standards and expectations that others have of them. Given the potential implications for people's health and wellbeing, **a lack of honesty and integrity by researchers is completely ethically unacceptable**.

Submitting a research proposal to an Ethics Committee

Seeking review of the ethical aspects of a study is highly recommended to reduce the risk of researchers making biased judgements regarding the consequences of their study. In addition, where research involves human subjects who will be recruited to a study through health service contacts, or where research will take place on health service property, it is vital that appropriate external ethical approval is acquired from the Local Research Ethics Committee (LREC).

Health-care research may need to be submitted to the LREC. If it is student research it may also need to be reviewed by an Ethics

Committee from an educational institute. LRECs work to national guidelines and look at the research submitted in terms of the welfare and dignity of participants and the validity of the research study. As an ethical review will take time, a researcher needs to contact the LREC administrator early on in the research process to find out the dates they will need to submit their proposal by, before they can start work. The student researcher needs to allow time to make any possible changes requested by the LREC. LRECs usually have a form that must be completed by the researcher. This covers the following information:

- Project title
- Name, details, experience and qualifications of the researcher (this includes the researcher's supervisor if this is a student application)
- Research objectives
- Outline of the research design
- Scientific background to the study
- Recruitment and sample details
- Tests, tools, devices and drugs to be used
- GP consent, if required
- Precautions to protect participants against potential discomfort, risk, breaches of confidentiality or the Data Protection Act
- Informed consent process (including consent forms and information sheets)
- Indemnity forms if drugs or equipment are to be used
- Likely costs and any sponsorship details

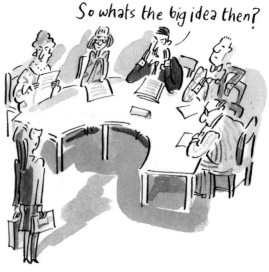

Ethics committees usually ask detailed questions to protect patients' interests, not to frighten researchers

Reflective activity

Considering ethical issues

Check your progress so far by working through each of the following questions. Write down your responses to each prompt to demonstrate that you have thought through the various ethical issues involved in conducting a research project.

1. What factors need to be taken into account to ensure that informed consent is gained from research participants?
2. What procedures can be put in place to protect confidentiality?
3. How can a researcher demonstrate honesty and integrity to participants and readers of a research study?

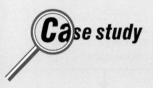 **Case study**

Andrew and the once-a-day insulin trial

Andrew has diabetes mellitus. Because of his inability to process glucose effectively, he has to inject himself with insulin twice a day. Andrew has been asked to be a participant in a randomised control trial of a new form of insulin that will only need to be administered once a day.

Patients in group A are to have two insulin injections. One will be a new, long-lasting insulin injection requiring once-a-day administration. The second will be a placebo injection. Group B are also going to receive two insulin injections. Both will be of normal insulin. Patients in both group A and group B will have their blood sugar monitored frequently (4-hourly).

Andrew would like to only have to inject his insulin once a day, so initially he feels he would like to be involved in the research study. If he is allocated to group B he may be using his usual type of insulin and having to monitor his blood sugar levels more frequently than he normally does. If he is allocated to group A he will still have to inject himself twice a day. Following the research study the new form of insulin may not be available for Andrew to use, even if he was receiving it and it was working effectively during the study.

Reflective activity

Consider the case study above.

1. Can this type of randomised controlled trial be viewed as unethical?
2. If Group A's treatment is better, is there an ethical problem in denying group B the benefits?
3. What issues would need to be considered to ensure that this research was ethical?
4. If you were in Andrew's place would you take part?
5. If you considered taking part, what questions would you like answered by the researcher?

Detailed planning and the research proposal

Before launching into data collection, professional and academic researchers usually produce a detailed plan of their intended research investigation. This is known as a *research proposal*. Many researchers have to produce one of these in order to obtain formal approval, or permission, to begin collecting data. Sometimes permission has to be sought from the people who are providing the money that will fund the study, or from an ethics committee that controls access to potentially vulnerable research participants, such as hospital patients. The research proposal outlines what the researchers wish to do, how they intend to go about it and what they hope to gain or achieve through the research investigation.

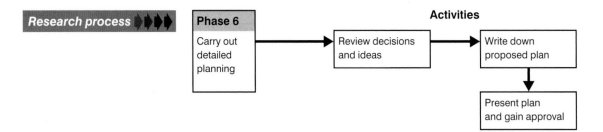

Figure 11.2 *Phase 6: Carry out detailed planning and gain ethical approval*

A lot of thinking and planning is undertaken before a researcher is in a position to produce a research proposal. It is useful for all researchers – and particularly for first-time researchers – to produce a research proposal even when there is no formal ethics committee or funding organisation involved. The research proposal ensures that the researcher has completed the required planning stages of the research process. Writing down the proposed plan in a detailed and explicit way helps researchers to think through, refine and express their research intentions.

It is usual, and advisable, to include a *schedule of work* with identified key dates in a plan at this stage. This may help researchers to realise that they need to rethink or redevelop certain parts of their intended project; for instance, gaining ethical approval and access to the research setting can be very time-consuming.

	September–October	October–November
Preparation phase	Preparation of research proposal/literature review	Gaining access/ethical approval
	December–February	**March–April**
Data phase	Data collection	Data analysis
	May–June	**July–August**
Writing phase	Analysis of research findings in relation to previous research	Preparation of the final report/thesis

Figure 11.3 *Example schedule of work – research proposal timetable*

Table 11.1 **A proposal form**
Answer each of the questions as fully as possible to describe the project that you propose to carry out
1. What is the title/topic area of your proposed research project?
2. What is the research question/hypothesis that you intend to investigate?
3. Explain why you have chosen to study this area and put forward this question/hypothesis
4. Where will you look for/find possible sources of background information on your chosen topic?
5. Who are your 'research population' going to be?
6. How will you identify a sample of people from the research population from whom to obtain data?
7. What different methods could you use to obtain data for your project?
8. How do you actually intend to obtain the data?
9. Why have you selected this/these method(s) rather than the others available?
10. What ethical issues do you need to be aware of in your research?
11. What will you do to ensure that you conduct 'ethically acceptable' research?
12. What problems/difficulties do you anticipate might occur in your research project?

Although the example of a work plan shows a linear route, some of the stages may run in parallel.

The research proposal also gives other people, such as the research supervisor, an opportunity to scrutinise the investigation plans and point out any weaknesses or obvious problems in it before approval to proceed is given. In some health-care courses, students may undertake development of a research proposal and submit this as their final assessment. They are not required to carry out the research but will have learnt a great deal about research from developing a cohesive research proposal.

A proposal can be set out in various ways. An example of a format that can be used to help researchers briefly outline their intentions is given in Table 11.1. Whatever structure is used for the research proposal the research ideas should be presented in a logical and clearly explained way. It can be helpful to follow the stages of the research process when doing this.

RRRRRRapid recap

Check your progress so far by working through each of the following questions.

1. What are the main ethical duties that should be considered before undertaking a research project?
2. If you were undertaking a student research project involving interviewing clinical staff from which groups should you seek ethical approval?
3. List the main headings required in a research proposal.

If you have difficulty with more than one of the questions, read through the section again to refresh your understanding before moving on.

Further reading

Central Office for Research Ethics Committees (COREC) (2002) Standard NHS REC application form. Available from: http://www.corec.org.ok.

Tod, A., Nicolson, P. and Allmark, P. (2002) Ethical review of health service research in the UK: implications for nursing. *Journal of Advanced Nursing*, **40**, 379–386.

World Medical Association (2000) *Declaration of Helsinki*, 5th amendment. http://www.wma.net/e/approvedhelsinki.html.

Analysing data

When a project has been adequately planned, a proposal has been written, ethical approval has been given and access has been agreed, a research study can begin. It is often best to begin the data collection stage of the research by running a pilot study.

Running a pilot study

A pilot study is a small trial run of an investigation to check out whether the procedures and methods that are intended to be used actually work. A pilot study may be run to test out a questionnaire, the experimental procedures or an observational technique.
The purpose of the pilot study is to identify any faults or weaknesses in the methods before they are used on a larger scale. The pilot study gives pointers that help the researcher to avoid problems and improve their intended data collection methods. Many first-time researchers also use a pilot study to gain confidence and develop their basic research technique before embarking on their larger-scale study.

A pilot study needs to be built in to the time schedule of the research investigation. However, care needs to be taken to ensure that you do not use up too much of your intended data source(s) during

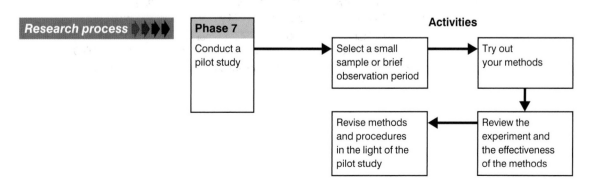

Figure 12.1 *Phase 7: Conduct a pilot study*

the pilot phase. It is best if you discard the data that you obtain in your pilot study rather than including it in any final analysis. Researchers do this because they often adjust their data collection tools as a result of the things that they learn from the pilot study. This means that they need to find new respondents for their full research project.

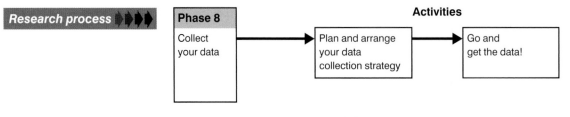

Figure 12.2 *Phase 8: Collect your data*

Making sense of the data

Once the required data has been obtained, the next task is to make sense of it. This process of making sense of data is usually referred to as *data analysis*. The way in which data analysis is done depends on the form(s) of data that are available. The obvious distinction that occurs is that data can take either a quantitative or qualitative form. It is possible that both forms of data will need to be analysed in a research study.

Data analysis takes quite a lot of time and needs to be planned into the research timetable in advance. Prior to data collection the researcher needs to decide how the data will be analysed. First-time researchers often underestimate this and assume that having collected data they have virtually finished their project. Data analysis is an involved and critical stage that still needs to be completed.

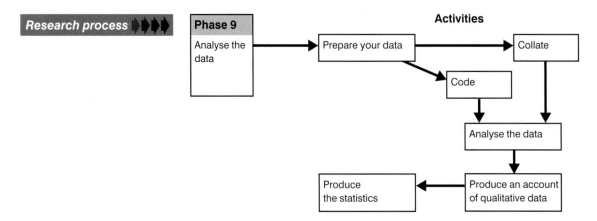

Figure 12.3 *Step 9: Analyse the data*

Analysing quantitative data

Quantitative data are numerical items of information. In analysing a set of quantitative data obtained in a small-scale student research study, some basic arithmetic may be used, and possibly some simple statistical techniques. Do not be put off by the idea of statistics. Even if you detest maths and feel threatened by numbers you should not fear statistics. Statistics are only a set of instruments or tools that are selected to help describe what is being studied. Statistics also enable the researcher to draw conclusions. In a small-scale research project you will only need to use basic descriptive statistics in your analysis of the quantitative data. If you understand what the different descriptive statistics tell you about the data, you will be able to clarify and discuss your findings.

Understanding the data

The process of analysing quantitative data basically involves counting and grouping together answers that are given to each closed question in a questionnaire, and counting and grouping into categories similar types of answer given to open questions. It is also possible to count and group observations that are made using participant observation

Table 12.1 **Analysing quantitative data**

Type of data	What does it involve?	Analysis possibilities
Nominal data (classificatory scales)	Nominal data are given a number to identify or code them. There is no natural numerical property to the data item, and it is not possible to measure the 'distance' between data items. For example, characteristics such as a person's sex, ethnicity and place of birth can all be given numerical codes	You can categorise and then count up the frequencies of each category in the data
Ordinal data (ranking scales)	These data are assigned numbers to indicate that there is an order or rank between them. For example, strongly agree = 5, agree = 4, no opinion = 3, disagree = 2, strongly disagree = 1. The data are not naturally numerical	You can use these data to produce frequencies and simple descriptive statistics
Interval data	These are recognised measurements, but there is no true zero. The start and end points of the measuring scale are arbitrary. However, the interval between the points on the scale is measurable. For example, temperature recordings provide interval data	Some basic descriptive statistics can be derived from this data
Ratio data	These are recognised measurements and have a true zero. Examples include money, age and measures of length and distance. For example, a person who is 20 years old is numerically twice as old as a child who is 10 years old	You can produce a variety of statistics from this type of data

and content analysis methods of data collection. The extent to which researchers are able to use statistical techniques (even basic ones) on their data and obtain useful information depends on the type of quantitative data with which they are working.

One problem that can occur in first-time research projects is that inexperience leads people to ask questions that produce only nominal data. This means that very little analysis of the data is possible. If lots of nominal data is produced, all that can be done is to count it up and *report* it. Ideally, the researcher should also be able to compare and contrast, so some ordinal data needs to also be collected and, ideally, interval and ratio data if possible.

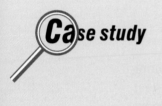

Joanne's research project

Joanne is doing a research project on the attitudes of midwives to women who smoke cigarettes during pregnancy. Her research question is 'Do the attitudes of midwives towards women who smoke cigarettes during pregnancy differ according to the length of time they have been qualified?' Her hypothesis is that midwives who have been qualified longer than 5 years are likely to be less critical of women who smoke cigarettes during pregnancy than midwives who have qualified within the last 5 years. She has decided to use a questionnaire to collect her data, and has written a number of questions in the hope of obtaining both quantitative and qualitative data.

Joanne asks respondents to indicate:

- Whether they are smokers or non-smokers
- Whether they strongly agree, agree, neither agree or disagree, disagree or strongly disagree with women smoking cigarettes during pregnancy
- How many cigarettes they themselves smoke each week
- Whether they have qualified as a midwife within the last 5 years

Data about whether a person is a smoker or non-smoker is nominal data. Answers have to be 'coded' to become numerical. Coding simply means creating numbered categories for responses and grouping similar responses together. *Smoker* may be coded '1' and *non-smoker* '2', for example. Joanne could then count up all of the 1's (or use a computer spreadsheet and get the analysis done automatically) and work out a very simple frequency distribution. This would tell her how many of the sample are smokers and how many are non-smokers. The only other thing that could be done with this data is to work out the *percentage* of respondents who fall into each category. You will probably see that this provides very little in the way of interesting data.

The same applies to all 'category' data (ethnicity, gender, age, religious affiliation and occupation, for example) that you collect. Be careful of putting all your quantitative eggs into the nominal basket!

Joanne's question on the extent to which respondents agree or disagree with women smoking during pregnancy offers more analysis possibilities. This is because it produces ordinal data. Again, the categories have to be coded to turn them into numerical items of information (strongly agree = 1, for example) but it is possible to make comparison between the categories. For example, she could compare the extent to which midwives qualifying in the last 5 years and those qualifying over 5 years ago agreed or disagreed with women smoking during pregnancy. She might even want to work out some percentages to describe the patterns in her data. If 80% of the more recently trained midwives were to disagree with women smoking during pregnancy compared to only 20% of those qualified over 5 years, Joanne might have the basis for an interesting discussion. What she couldn't say at this point is that length of qualification is the primary influence on midwives' attitudes to women who smoke during pregnancy. Joanne does not have the data to support this assertion.

In response to a question about how many cigarettes they smoke each week, respondents would give Joanne an actual numerical answer (for example, 'five cigarettes a week'). This is ratio data. There is a true zero figure and the numbers given can be organised into genuine ranked categories (0–5, 6–10 and so on). This true numerical data opens up lots of possibilities for statistical analysis.

Preparing quantitative data for analysis

The first stage of quantitative data analysis involves actually preparing the data to get it into an 'analysable' form. The two things that need to be done with quantitative data are:

- Coding the responses or observation categories
- Collating them into a table of responses.

The main method of collecting quantitative data in student research is usually through the use of questionnaires. Most student questionnaires feature a mixture of 'open' and 'closed' questions. Closed questions generally produce quantitative data and are relatively easy to code. We will look at coding the findings from 'open' questions in the section on analysing qualitative data below.

Imagine that you are conducting a survey on nurses' attitudes to nurse–patient relationships and that you are using a questionnaire to collect data on aspects of this topic. Your first two questions require some basic demographic information, while the third and fourth questions seek data on 'patient relationships'.

Example

Nurses' attitudes to nurse–patient relationships

Question	Code	Type of data
1. What sex are you?		
Male	(1)	Nominal data
Female	(2)	
2. How old are you (years only)?		
18–20	(1)	Ratio data
21–23	(2)	
24–26	(3)	
27–29	(4)	
30+	(5)	
3. Choose **one** response that most clearly matches your view of the statement below		
'Nurses should try not to get too closely involved with their patients'		
I strongly agree	(1)	Ordinal data
I agree	(2)	
I neither agree or disagree	(3)	
I disagree	(4)	
I strongly disagree	(5)	
4. Describe the characteristics of an ideal nurse–patient relationship:		

You will note that the first three questions are 'coded'; that is, the potential answers have all been given a code number in advance. When the researcher has collected all the data they need, the next step is to produce a table of coded responses (Table 12.2).

You should code all the 'closed questions' and fixed response items in your questionnaire in advance of collecting any data. You can then just circle the response code that matches your respondent's answer as you work through, asking the questions. When you have collected all your data, simply enter the response codes into a coding sheet such as this one. Ideally, do this on a computer spreadsheet (or transfer your data to one) as the program will calculate a variety of simple statistics for you.

Table 12.2 **An example of answers given by five respondents to the first three questions above**			
Question	**1**	**2**	**3**
Person A	1	1	2
Person B	2	4	1
Person C	2	4	1
Person D	1	3	3
Person E	2	2	1

Making sense of quantitative data

'Analysis' means separating something that is 'whole' into its component parts so that it can be studied. The 'whole' data set needs to be separated into its component parts in order to find meaningful patterns and relationships in the mass of data that has been accumulated. Once the data has been prepared, it can be analysed by applying a number of simple descriptive statistics techniques. The basic techniques that will looked at here are:

● Frequency distributions

● Mean, median and mode

● Standard deviations

These are all forms of *descriptive statistics*. They provide a summary of the pattern of information that can be found in a sample. These statistics do not say anything about whether the patterns in the data are likely to apply in, or can be generalised to, the population as a whole.

How to produce a frequency distribution

A frequency distribution is a simple tally of how often (or frequently) certain data items occur within a data set. Frequency distributions are used to give simple descriptive information about the variables in a set of data. To produce a frequency distribution, simply total up the number of each type of response given to a particular question or the number of each type of observation that is made. You can then use these numbers to produce a frequency table (see the table in the example overleaf), a bar chart (Figure 12.4) or a pie chart (Figure 12.5).

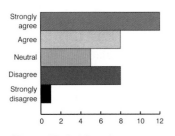

Figure 12.4 *A bar chart.*

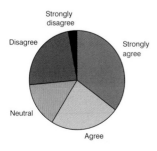

Figure 12.5 *A pie chart.*

Example

'Nurses should be payed higher salaries' – a frequency table

	Code	Number	%
Strongly agree	1	12	35
Agree	2	8	23.5
Neutral	3	5	15
Disagree	4	8	23.5
Strongly disagree	5	1	3
Total		**34**	**100**

Calculating the mean, median and mode

The mean, median and mode are measures of *central tendency*. The *mean* is the numerical value around which the data is centred. Researchers calculate means in their data sets to get an idea of 'average' values. The mean is easy to calculate (see the accompanying box). If data items collected are not numerical there can still be a need to know what the most common or midpoint items are. The *mode* is the most frequently occurring data item. The *median* is the value of the midpoint in a data set. The following example box illustrates these three simple, descriptive forms of central tendency.

Calculating the standard deviation

The mean shows only where the numerical average is within a data

---

Example

Dietary supplements reportedly eaten by a group of 20 patients over a 2-day period

0, 0, 1, 1, 1, 2, 3, 3, 4, 5, 5, 6, 7, 7, 8, 8, 8, 9, 9, 25

Mean = total number of supplements/number of patients = 6

Median = number of supplements eaten by the patient at the midpoint of the set, i.e. the 10th/11th = 5

Mode = the number of supplements eaten by the most patients = 8

---

distribution. The standard deviation is a measure that shows how much the data varies from the mean. Knowing how much *dispersion* or spread there is around the mean can be helpful in assessing the extent to which your respondents are similar or different. For example, if most respondents said that they strongly agreed that nurses' wages should be higher, you would get a low standard deviation and be

Example

Let us work out the standard deviation of the data set collected from our dietary supplement patients

Step 1: The mean of the data set is 6

Step	2	3
Item	Deviation	Square of deviation
0	− 6	36
0	− 6	36
1	− 5	25
1	− 5	25
1	− 5	25
2	− 4	16
3	− 3	9
3	− 3	9
4	− 2	4
5	− 1	1
5	− 1	1
6	0	0
7	+1	1
7	+1	1
8	+2	4
8	+2	4
8	+2	4
9	+3	9
9	+3	9
25	+19	361

Step 4:
Sum of squares = 580

Step 5:
Variance (sum of squares ÷ number of items)
= 580 ÷ 20 = 29

Step 6:
Square root of variance
= 5.385
= standard deviation (SD)

aware from this that they generally felt much the same. To calculate the standard deviation you need to:

1. Calculate the mean of the data set
2. Calculate the difference, or 'deviation', between each individual response and the mean value; if the difference is higher it will produce a plus (positive) figure, and if it is lower it will produce a minus (negative) figure
3. Calculate the square of each of these 'deviations'
4. Add the squared figures together to get a 'sum of squares' figure
5. Divide the sum of squares by the number of data items to get a 'variance' figure
6. Calculate the square root of the variance figure to obtain the standard deviation.

The standard deviation from the mean of 5.385 is relatively low. This suggests that the mean is quite a good representation of the average amount of dietary supplements taken by the respondents over the 2-day period. Please note also that, because of the relatively small number of items in the calculation, the standard deviation in our example is statistically questionable. It is just used here for illustrative purposes.

Statistical tests

No one is expected to quote statistical formulae that make up a statistical test, or explain the intricacies of how they work. The important thing is to know which type of test to apply (with the guidance of your research supervisor) and when not to apply a statistical test. A lot of statistical analysis is concerned with looking at data against a set of expectations and making decisions about the difference. If an experimental or quasi-experimental approach to a research area has been taken the researcher and the reader of the research report will need to find out if the results were due to chance. If the difference cannot be considered to be due to chance this is termed a *statistically significant* result. In other words, how probable is it that the results are due to the introduction of the independent variable, or are they due to a chance happening or one or two extreme cases affecting the data?

Probability refers to whether an event is likely to occur. For instance, if you toss a coin 100 times you would expect it to land heads up around 50 times out of the 100. In statistical terms this would be expressed as a decimal = 0.5. The probability (p) would be 0.5 (or 50%). Working out the likely probability of a particular result occurring from a coin toss is relatively straightforward. However, researchers often face more complicated scenarios where they need to make a judgement about the likelihood of their findings being the result of chance. How can they judge this likelihood?

To assess (and limit) the influence of chance on their findings, researchers calculate and report their findings in terms of 'levels of significance'. Usually a significance level of either 0.05 (5%) or 0.01 (1%) is chosen and the result is tested against this. This means that, if the findings of a particular event would only have arisen by chance less than 5% of the time, then chance is rejected as a possible explanation for the results if they are statistically significant at a level of 0.05%. In other words, the chances of these findings occurring by accident are less than 5 in 100.

Many statistical tests are available to determine the probability and statistical significance of research findings. Some of the tests available are appropriate with particular types of numerical data and cannot be applied in all situations. It is beyond the scope of this book to look in detail at all the statistical tests. The main names and types of statistical test are listed here. If the data requires a statistical test this may be done using a statistical computing package or in some instances the researcher may be able to undertake the calculations using the statistical formula. The formulae and how to do these calculations will not be explained here; however, if you wish to undertake statistical tests in your research, the further reading at the end of this chapter should be consulted. Student researchers should always seek research statistics advice before starting their data collection, as the form of analysis needs to be decided before data is collected.

Tests for categories (nominal data)

As previously discussed, nominal data involves categories. Nominal data are given a number to identify or code them. There is no natural numerical property to the data item, and it is not possible to measure the 'distance' between data items. For example, characteristics such as a person's sex, ethnicity and place of birth can all be given numerical codes.

Three types of test are used to identify whether the results from nominal data are statistically significant:

- Chi-squared (χ^2) test: used when there is only one classification or category
- Cross-tabulation test: used when there are two classifications or categories
- Log-linear analysis: used if there are more than two classifications or categories.

Table 12.3 **Statistical tests for measurements (ordinal, interval or ratio)**			
Associations between variables	**Number of variables**	**Differences between groups**	**Number of groups**
Pearson correlation	2	't' test	2
Spearman correlation	More than 2	Wilcoxon test	2
Multiple regression	More than 2	Mann–Whitney test	2
		Anova test	More than 2
		Friedman test	More than 2
		Kruskal–Wallis test	More than 2

The tests identified in Table 12.3 ('tests for measurements') show some of the wide range of statistical tests that can be applied to ordinal, interval and ratio data. All of the tests identified here are used to determine associations or differences between variables or groups. The decision to use a particular test is part of a whole process of determining the *statistical inference*. That is, working out what can be reasonably claimed about the results by the use of statistics.

Presenting numerical data

Key points / **Top tips**

Where do you put statistical data in a research report?

● Statistical tables that highlight particularly interesting findings are usually put in the main body of the text, close to where the content is discussed. In such cases the full statistical tables, from which the smaller tables have been derived, should be placed at the end of the report.

The numerical findings contained within a research report are usually presented in a format that helps the reader understand the information 'at a glance'. Any statistical tests applied to the data need to be identified with the data being presented. Tables are the most basic way of presenting numerical data or written information. Throughout this book tables have been used to present information, such as the advantages and disadvantages of particular types of data collection tool. It is important to label all rows and columns, and accurately title the table. You have already seen two other examples of ways of presenting data in the form of the bar chart (Figure 12.4) and the pie chart (Figure 12.5). Bar charts are a popular way of presenting simple data such as quantities or numbers under different descriptive categories. Both axes need to be clearly labelled within a report and should have a relevant and informative title. Pie charts are a really useful way of showing the relative proportions of different categories within a survey.

Reflective activity

Look through research articles and locate one in which a **line graph** has been used to present data. Line graphs involve a series of points plotted on a graph that are then joined together to make a line. In your chosen article, what was it about the data that made a line graph the most useful way of presenting it?

Line graphs are typically used to show changes in quantities or trends over time. For example, they are often used in epidemiological studies that show the rate of increase of a particular disease over time.

Analysing qualitative data

Data collection methods such as participant observation and in-depth interviews allow less control over the type and range of information that respondents give than methods such as questionnaires. Responses to 'open' questions and observation of 'natural' behaviour are hard to predict. Words – expressing attitudes and opinions, for example – rather than numbers, are the 'units of analysis' produced by qualitative research methods. Both of these factors can cause problems for researchers when it comes to making sense of the qualitative data that they have obtained. The stages involved in analysing qualitative data are identified here.

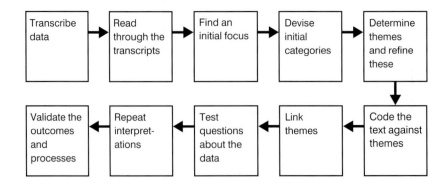

Figure 12.6 *Stages in analysing qualitative data (Wood 2001, p. 89)*

Preparing qualitative data for analysis

As with quantitative data, the first thing that you need to do with your qualitative data is to prepare it for analysis. The two key steps of coding and collating data are again helpful to follow. The difference when working with qualitative data is that the useful items of information are usually a part of a much larger body of information, most of which is not useful with regard to your research question.

One of the strategies that researchers use to 'capture' data during interviews is to tape-record what the respondent says during conversation. This ensures that the researcher gets a verbatim, or word-for-word, account, but it also has implications in that the researcher may have to transcribe the interview ('write out' what was said). Transcribing can be very time-consuming. Some researchers find this valuable, as they learn a lot about their data by doing it, while others conclude that wholesale transcribing of interviews is best avoided. Researchers get around the problem of wholesale transcribing by listening to their tapes repeatedly, and using the 'pause' button to allow them to transcribe the most interesting and useful sections. This is one way of beginning the process of coding data. Remember to assess the data in terms of whether it is relevant to your research question.

If you have interviews on a specific topic with several people, or if you have observed a number of similar situations, it is likely that there will be patterns, themes and similarities in the data. Your analysis task is to find them. You need to decide on some theme or pattern categories (give them a name) and allocate data items to these. You will need to read through all your data and assess the 'meaning' of each answer. This requires a careful and sensitive approach to the data, so that you retain the 'meaning' that the respondents intended to give in their responses.

Not all answers will fit neatly into your categories. As a result, you will need to make some judgements about how to deal with these items – and should acknowledge this.

Making sense of qualitative data

Analysing qualitative data is usually quite an involved and time-consuming process. This is largely because you first have to organise the data into a manageable format. You may have questionnaires with written answers of various lengths to open questions. Alternatively, you may have tape-recorded your respondents' answers to interview questions and have a great deal of tape to listen to. Whatever form the data happens to be in, you will need to reorganise it.

Let us imagine that your qualitative data consists of written responses to three open questions. How can you analyse it? The first step is to make a copy of the original data. You should always keep your original, full data set to refer back to if you need to. Work with the copy. In this situation it would be best to collect together the responses to each question. You might want to cut the relevant sections out of the copied questionnaires. You then need to read the responses several times, thinking about possible similarities between them that could justify grouping them into distinct categories. It is best to do this several times, learning from the data as you do so. Look for themes and patterns all the time. As you can probably imagine, this does take some time and mental effort.

When you have identified themes and patterns, you need to describe them, and perhaps use direct quotes as examples, in a discussion of your findings. You may also want to try to convert some of the qualitative data into a quantitative form to give you further detail to discuss. Having interpreted the data it is advisable to take your findings back to the people being studied for respondent validation to check that they have confidence in your interpretation.

Presenting qualitative data

Quantitative data is usually presented in statistical and graphical formats. It is relatively easy to present because it is numerical. On the other hand, qualitative data is not so straightforward, and requires a more word-based style of presentation. Qualitative data is usually presented as a written discussion. Researchers tend to make use of short verbatim quotes of what respondents said or wrote. They do this to provide evidence of typical or particularly important responses and statements. These are often used to clarify and illustrate the key themes and patterns in the data. In addition to describing and reporting on key themes that are found within the data, qualitative researchers also tend to comment on what was different between respondents, or what was lacking from the data.

While most qualitative research reports depend on written discussions of findings, it is also possible to make use of other devices, such as images, tape recordings, diagrams and flow charts. These can be used to communicate and provide evidence of the key findings. Whatever method is used, the validity of the data should always be preserved.

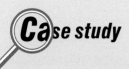

Case study

Example of qualitative data transcribed in full

Participant: You see I … in many ways I like it because I think … to say that we give holistic care means that we have got to have a finger in every pot and I think that is exactly what we have got because I think you do give holistic care because we are the co-ordinators so we have we are involved in every single part every aspect of what's going on with the patient having said that it is very difficult where you've also got a nursing role as well it is so difficult to split all your time

Researcher: Do you find that it is increasing? I've described it as a pivotal role there's all these different people coming with information about this one client or whatever and then you've got this management of nursing. Do you find that those that trying to do the nursing and organise that conflicting with the umm other role?

Participant: I don't think it's umm I think … I think that skill mix has a huge effect on this because umm a few months ago when our skill mix was different we were still trying to do this and the staff nurses were working hours over their shifts and it was very difficult because we were doing both and we wouldn't let them conflict …… a slight change in skill mix on the ward which has increased the number of trained staff actually at the moment is allowing us to do it quite nicely and I don't think they do conflict at all because umm …… it it's tremendous to know everything that's going on with that patient and we do and it helps our nursing to do it because we can tailor their day and the care that they're being given by the nurses by knowing exactly what's going on with every single you know discipline so I think at the end of the day when you think about it the nurses spend probably 90% of the day with the patients these people just come in and out we are the people that need to do all you know to know it I mean we need to be the people that are organising it

Researcher: Umm having said that though obviously it's only as good as the relationships that the trained staff have with doctors etc. do you find that a time-consuming thing are relationships ever strained with that?

Participant: Umm …… I think that yeah I think it is a time-consuming thing but I think it's something that reaps benefits so we as a group of nurses … have actually gone out of our way to develop these relationships with people because we feel we get more out of it than we actually put into it eventually so things that we have decided to do like … invite the OT, the social worker once a week to come and sit with us and talk to us get to know us umm I mean we are on first name terms with all of our the multidisciplinary team, we ring people up and we use their first names and we can get favours done we can get all of these … you can get a lot of help and I think … it is time-consuming but I find that it actually stops conflict because if you can reason with somebody and say now come on you know you know we don't do that normally and we know this hasn't been done in this case but you know that that doesn't happen on here and they you know it really does help and when there's an awful lot of conflict between the medical staff and nurses I think … there's not so much conflict with the other multidisciplinary team members

RRRRRRapid recap

Check your progress so far by working through each of the following questions.

1. When do you code data ready for analysis?
2. What sorts of basic descriptive statistical techniques can be applied to quantitative data?
3. How does a researcher prepare qualitative data for analysis?
4. How are quantitative findings usually presented?

If you have difficulty with more than one of the questions, read through the section again to refresh your understanding before moving on.

Reference

Wood, N (2001) *The health project book: a handbook for new researchers in the field of health*. Routledge, London.

Further reading

Armitage, P. and Berry, G. (1994) *Statistical Methods in Medical Research*, 3rd edn. Blackwell Scientific, Oxford.

Bowers, D. (1996) *Statistics From Scratch: An introduction for health care professionals*. John Wiley, Chichester.

Coffey, A. and Atkinson, P. (1996) *Making Sense of Qualitative Data*. Sage, Thousand Oaks, CA.

Gissane, C. (1998) Understanding and using descriptive statistics. *British Journal of Occupational Therapy*, **61**, 267–272.

Savage, J. (2000) One voice, different tunes: issues raised by dual analysis of a segment of qualitative data. *Journal of Advanced Nursing*, **31**, 1493–1500.

Writing a research report

Learning outcomes

By the end of this chapter you should be able to:

● Identify an appropriate structure for a research report
● Reference consistently within a research report
● Appreciate the need for dissemination of research findings

Writing up a research report is one of the last stages of completing a research investigation. The report should be written in a way that communicates both the *process* (what the researcher did) and the *findings* (what they discovered) to people who read it.

Nurses and other health-care practitioners sometimes complain that research is not put into practice because the research reports are not easy to understand and sufficiently interesting to read. The established way of doing this is to follow a commonly used research report structure. Research reports generally follow this common structure because it enables:

● Researchers to outline their research investigation and findings in a logical sequence
● Readers to focus on key features of the research without having to read the whole report
● Readers to critique research reports more easily
● Other researchers to make comparisons with similar research investigations
● Researchers to guard against writing a biased account due to their personal views and feelings.

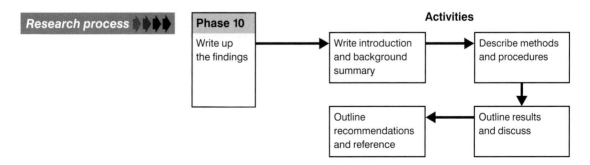

Figure 13.1 *Phase 10: Write up the findings*

A report should not develop haphazardly. During its early stages, five questions need to be considered and should be kept in mind throughout

- What is the report for? (purpose)
- What should it include? (content)
- Who is it written for? (audience)
- What structure should the report take? (shape)
- How should it be written? (language)

Purpose A research report does not just make findings available, it also allows people not to make similar mistakes or to replicate similar methods used.

Content A research report should include justification or discussion about all important research decisions, including ethical implications.

Shape A research report needs to group material into sections or chapters presented in a logical way and of an appropriate length. Statistical data that are particularly interesting are usually put within the main body of the text. The full statistical data available can be placed at the end of the report. References to the full tables can be made in the text so that the reader can consult them if they wish to.

Audience A piece of research may be written up several times in different ways, for different people – for example, specialists reading technical journals, people mainly interested from an application to practice perspective and the general public. The audience determines the language chosen for the report.

Language Every subject has its own language, and this is true of research. Throughout this book research terms have been explained because there is a need to strike a balance between 'writing over the heads of' and 'writing down to' the readers.

Constructing a research report

A standard research report structure is described below, with some guidance on the content of each section.

The title

The title should be informative and should refer closely and descriptively to the focus of the research. The title page should also contain the researcher's name.

O—π *Keywords*

Abstract
It is easier to read something if you are aware at the start of what it is about. Authors of research reports attract the reader by giving a summary of the study and the main results at the start of a report.

The abstract

An **abstract** is a short summary (100–200 words) of the investigation with 'thumbnail' details, including the aims, methods and main conclusions. Some researchers refer to this as the 'rationale' section of the report. The abstract should be able to stand on its own as a succinct and intelligible summary of the entire report. A clear abstract encourages people to read the entire report. It is often the last task to be completed when writing up the research report.

The introduction

The introduction explains the rationale for the research, summarises background reading about previous work in the same area and explains the aims, research question(s) and hypothesis (if there is one) of the research. The goal here is to establish a clear logic, building from a description and analysis of previous research, background information and theory to a statement of the specific purpose of the research project.

Method

The 'method' section outlines how the researcher went about the research study. A description of the methods should enable readers to assess the objectivity of the research and whether appropriate ethical standards were adopted. The goal here is to describe the data sources (for example, the sample), the data collection tools that were used and the procedures that were undertaken to collect the data. The explanation should be clear enough for another person to be able to repeat and conduct the study in the same way.

For ease of reading the 'method' section is often subdivided into three parts:

- **Data sources**. If people were the key data source, the main demographic characteristics of the population are identified (sex, age and so on). If the data were obtained from an analysis of texts, TV programmes or some other inanimate source, the key characteristics or identifiers of those sources need to be described. The total sample size, the criteria and method used to select sample members or items, or the case study situation, and any criteria used to exclude others should be clearly discussed.

- **The 'methodology' section**. Identifies the method(s) that were used to collect the data. Any questionnaires, observation records or other data collection tools are described. A full, blank copy of these tools should be included in the appendix at the end of the report.

- **The 'procedure' section**. This should include a step-by-step account of how the data were collected. The conditions under which participants were interviewed or observed should be referred to, as well as the specific instructions given to participants. If a questionnaire or other research tool has been used, an explanation of how it was administered should be given.

Findings

The findings of the research are presented in an appropriate statistical, graphical or written form. Raw data does not need to be included in the main body of the report. At this point, the findings should be described without any further analysis or comment.

Discussion and conclusions

In the 'discussion' section the findings are examined in terms of the patterns, points of interest and conclusions that they lead the researcher to draw. The researcher must be careful to ensure that any conclusions are actually supported by the data that have been obtained. In this section it is useful if the findings are compared and contrasted to findings from other similar studies, and with existing theories. The researcher should critically evaluate the validity of the findings and the extent to which they provide answers to the research questions, indicate whether the findings support or refute the hypothesis, and comment on the reliability of the data.

Recommendations

Researchers often wish to recommend ways in which the research could be extended or modified to develop or extend knowledge and understanding of the area on which the report was focusing.

References

All the sources of information that are used in a research report must be referenced. The listing should be alphabetical and should follow a standard referencing system so that the source can be traced.

Appendices

These contain material that is integral to the research, such as a copy of the questionnaire or research/interview notes. While any researcher should keep their original, raw data in case an independent reviewer wishes to see it, it is not usual practice to include it anywhere in the final research report.

Some dangers to be aware of when writing a final report

- Do not under-estimate the time and effort required for writing up a report – about one-third of the total time for doing the research will be taken up in writing the report
- Do not over-estimate the readers' background knowledge of your topic
- Do not use long, rambling sentences or explanations; write simply and clearly
- Do not use too many 'I' statements – 'I did this, and then I found that' is best avoided; focus on the topic and the data
- Do not pad out your report with irrelevant information or pictures
- Keep to the word limit if the research is part of a course of study

There is no need to worry if the hypothesis is not supported by the research findings. Researchers should not falsify the findings or become less objective in analysis in order to avoid saying that the hypothesis was not supported. The important thing is that the research is conducted and analysed correctly. The researcher and reader can then both identify when the hypothesis is not supported by the data. This is perfectly acceptable, and is in no way 'wrong' or incorrect.

Referencing within a research report

One of the final tasks that researchers have to undertake when 'writing up' is to check that they have correctly referenced all the books, articles and other data sources that are referred to in the report. If a complete and accurate record of the sources that were used during the background information search and throughout the research process is kept this should make the reference list in the final report easier to compile. If not the, researcher has to trace the details of all the sources they have used before they can move on.

There are a number of standardised referencing techniques that are used by academic and professional researchers. Most journals that publish research reports indicate which referencing system they want authors to use. Mainly a researcher just needs to choose one and use it correctly and consistently. The Harvard system and the Vancouver system are referencing methods that are commonly used in research publications. Under the Harvard system:

- References are cited in the main text of the report by including the author's surname followed by the year of publication in brackets; for example, Walsh (2000)
- Where there are two authors, include them in the text as, surname and surname (year); for example, Millar and Rogers (2000)
- Where there are more than two authors, insert the first author's surname and then use *et al.* (short for the Latin *et alii*, meaning 'and others'); for example, Johnson *et al.* (2000)
- Direct quotations must be in quotation marks, followed by the author's surname, the year of publication and the page number of the reference (in brackets); for example, 'representativeness refers to the question of whether the group or situation being studied are typical of others' (McNeill 1990:87)
- References are listed in alphabetical order at the end of the text, in the same way as in the Further Reading section on page 132.

A journal example using the Harvard system is:

Waring, T. (1996) Prisoners with diabetes: do they receive appropriate care? *Nursing Times*, **92**, 38–39.

A book example using the Harvard system is:

Parkes, C. and Weiss, R. (1983) *Recovery from Bereavement*. Basic Books, New York.

Under the Vancouver system:

- References are numbered (number in brackets) consecutively through the text
- Each reference is then listed in numerical order at the end of the text
- Journals are assigned standard abbreviations from *Index Medicus*, the American National Library of Medicine's catalogue of terms and abbreviations.

A journal example of a Vancouver reference is:

Waring T. Prisoners with diabetes: do they receive appropriate care? *Nursing Times 1996*; 92: 38–39.

A book reference example using the Vancouver system is:

Parkes C, Weiss R. *Recovery from Bereavement*. New York: Basic Books, 1983.

Reflective activity

Using referencing systems

Use the Harvard system to correctly reference each of the following:

1. An article from *Nursing Times* (pp. 36–38) called 'Treating obesity in people with learning disabilities', by Michael Perry. August 1996, Volume 92, issue 35.

2. A paper entitled 'Pakistani women and maternity care: raising muted voices', written by A. M. Bowes and T. Meehan Domokos, appeared in vol. 18, no. 1, 1996, pages 45–65 of the journal *Sociology of Health and Illness*.

3. An author called Steven Pryjmachuk had a paper published in July 1996 entitled, 'Adolescent schizophrenia: families' information needs'. It was in *Mental Health Nursing* vol. 16, no. 4.

4. A book published in 1996 by Open University Press, Buckingham, by Loraine Blaxter, Christine Hughes and Malcolm Tight, called 'How to Research'.

Key points **Top tips**

Writing up a research report

- Follow convention: use a standard report structure in your 'write up'
- It is easier to write the abstract last (if you are using one)
- Show clearly how your conclusions are supported by the data that you have collected
- Try to offer some constructive criticism of your own research process and findings – nobody's research is perfect, and you will show greater understanding by pointing out the weaknesses and limitations of yours
- Remember to say whether your findings support or refute the original hypothesis, or how they answer the initial research question
- Reference your work fully and accurately.
- Check that the spelling and grammar are correct. Word processing programmes can help you to do this. However, do not rely totally on spell-checkers. You should still proof-read your work afterwards to cheque for odd errors that the spell-checker overlooks!
- Word processing is a good way of ensuring that your work is neatly presented.

Disseminating the research findings

At the start of the book the research process was described as having 10 phases – well, perhaps it is advisable to add a further very important step of *research dissemination*. The word dissemination means to 'spread widely', and research dissemination involves the purposeful communication of research findings. Health-care practitioners who have undertaken small-scale studies may be reluctant to disseminate their findings because they cannot be generalised. However, if the limitations of the research are clearly reported there should not be a reluctance to circulate the report. Too much health-care research sits on shelves after a huge amount of work has gone into undertaking it.

There are many methods of dissemination of research. These include:

- Summaries of the key points circulated locally
- Conferences – presentations, seminars and posters
- Research workshops
- Local and national journal publications.

Student health-care practitioners can, at the least, present their findings to the other group members. Although dissemination of a piece of research alone does not guarantee that it will be used, just by making the research available the researcher has tried to break down the barrier of the inaccessibility. Research must be accessible. Even if you do not undertake research yourself, you have hopefully grasped through using this book that research is not an alien thing, and that it can affect everyday health and social-care practice.

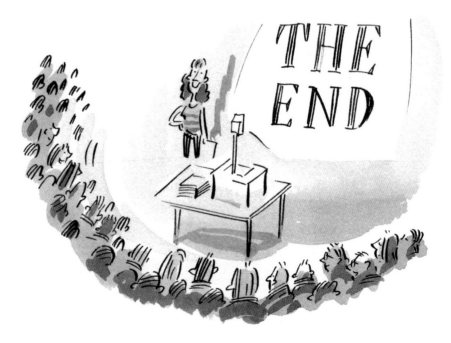

Finally presenting your completed research report can be satisfying and exciting (as well as a little bit scary)

ʀʀʀʀʀ*Rapid recap*

Check your progress so far by working through each of the following questions.

1. What are the main sections that should be contained in a research report?
2. Identify three possible 'dangers' in writing up a research report.
3. Through what routes can the findings from a research study be disseminated?

If you have difficulty with more than one of the questions, read through the section again to refresh your understanding before moving on.

Reference

McNeill, P. (1990) *Research Methods*. Routledge, London.

Further reading

Hamill, C. (1999) Academic essay writing in the first person: a guide for undergraduates. *Nursing Standard*, **13**, 38–40.

Appendix

Rapid Recap – answers

Chapter 1

1. **Give three terms that describe research and indicate the difference between research and other forms of knowledge.**

   Research is (a) controlled, (b) rigorous and (c) systematic. Knowledge gained from research is usually valued more highly than non-research based knowledge.

2. **Explain what the term 'epistemology' means.**

   The theory of knowledge – i.e., how we know what we do.

3. **Jot down the different stages of the research process.**

   Phases of the research process:

   1. Identify a topic of interest
   2. Obtain and review background information
   3. Identify a research question or hypothesis
   4. Choose a research strategy and design
   5. Choose data collection methods
   6. Carry out detailed planning and gain ethical and other clearance to collect data
   7. Conduct a pilot study
   8. Collect your data
   9. Analyse the data
   10. Write up the findings.

Chapter 2

1. **How does evidence-based practice differ from simply using the findings of a research study in practice?**

   As it is rare for a single research study to offer a definite answer to a question, and some even prove inconclusive, evidence-based practice allows us to combine the findings from several in order to improve practice.

2. **Why is it sometimes difficult to get research findings used to improve practice?**

   Different research studies asking the same question might provide us with different, indeed conflicting, answers. This makes it difficult to implement their results in practice.

3. **What does the term 'clinical audit' mean?**

   Clinical audit uses methods rather like research and examines whether the best existing knowledge is really informing what is actually occurring in practice.

Chapter 3

1. **What is the difference between pure and applied research?**

   Pure research is conceptual and focuses on developing and testing abstract theories. Applied research applies theories and research methods to real situations.

2. **What does descriptive research set out to do?**

   To extend knowledge through painting a mental picture of the findings from the systematic collection and recording of data.

3. **What are researchers who conduct correlation research looking for?**

   They aim to establish links between two factors (variables) within the research.

4. **What kind of research asks 'How' and 'Why' questions?**

   Explanatory research.

5. **Can you give two examples of secondary data sources that a researcher might use?**

   Newspaper articles and patients' case notes.

6. **How does primary data differ from secondary data?**

   Primary data is data collected by researchers themselves, whereas secondary data already exists.

7. **What term would be used to describe numerical information obtained by a researcher?**

   Quantitative data.

Chapter 4

1. **If a researcher is gathering data using a structured questionnaire that allows numerical analysis, what is the likely theoretical approach adopted for the research?**

   The researcher would probably use the positivist approach.

2. **A researcher is collecting data through observing biology lecturers teaching on health-care courses as they go about their everyday work. What is the likely theoretical approach underpinning this research?**

   The researcher would probably use the naturalistic approach.

3. **Identify the difference between the terms theory testing and theory building.**

   Theory testing means to build on existing theories, exploring and developing them; theory building means to identify new theories.

Chapter 5

1. **Name two things that weaken the reliability of a data collection method.**

   a) The researcher working alone

   b) Collecting the data in a situation that cannot be replicated.

2. **What does the concept of validity refer to?**

   Whether the data collected is a true picture of what is being studied.

3. **Why cannot you assume that interview data is 100% valid?**

   Because the respondents may not answer truthfully.

4. **Explain why some researchers try to ensure that they select a representative sample of people for their research studies.**

   If researchers ensure that they select a representative sample of people for their studies, they can feel more confident in generalising the findings.

5. **What are you if you are not objective?**

   If you are not objective, you are letting your values and beliefs influence the way in which you develop a project. You are said to be biased or prejudiced.

6. **What is termed the 'gold standard' of evidence-based practice?**

   Randomised control trials.

7. **What is the difference between a systematic review and a clinical guideline?**

   A systematic review is a summary of all the available research evidence on a given area, using a rigorous approach across many research studies. Clinical guidelines are tools developed using the best available evidence at the time, offering recommendations for practice in a given situation.

Chapter 6

Answers will depend on student's choice of research study.

Chapter 7

1. **Give two reasons for undertaking a background literature review before starting a research study.**

   a) To clarify the problem/hypothesis

   b) To increase understanding of the topic area, and what research has been done already.

2. **Identify as many possible sources for background literature that a researcher could access.**

   Textbooks, journals, magazines and newspapers, CD-ROM, Internet, organisations.

Chapter 8

1. **What does the term critical evaluation mean?**

   The systematic reading of a research article or report and the subsequent balanced commentary on it.

2. **What are the four main stages in constructing a research critique?**

   a) Read the research report critically

   b) Examine the methods

   c) Be critical

   d) Write the critique.

3. **Why is having the ability to critique research a useful skill for health-care practitioners?**

   Because, without that skill, they might change their practice as a result of reading the report of a research study that has serious flaws.

Chapter 9

1. **Why is random sampling a useful method for choosing a research group from a large population?**

   A random sample is likely to give a representative research group to study with similar characteristics to the large population. If the sample is large enough this will then allow researchers to generalise their findings.

2. **What is the role of a 'control group' in an experimental study?**

   To allow the researcher to compare the data from the experimental group and decide whether the findings are due to the experimental variable.

3. **Could an in-depth single interview with a patient be described as a case study?**

   Yes, it could well be a case study. The methods used to gain access to the patient for the interview, data collection techniques, analysis and presentation of findings would determine whether or not this was case study research.

Chapter 10

1. **What is the difference between a cross-sectional study design and a before-and-after research design?**

   A cross-sectional study design is a simple 'snapshot', at a particular time, of what is being studied. A before-and-after research design is used to measure the extent to which the subject under study has changed. This type of research is really two cross-sectional studies conducted on the same subject at different moments in time.

2. **If you were researching the need for dietary supplements for elderly patients while hospitalised, what would be the advantages and disadvantages of the following data collection methods?**

   - Questionnaire
   - Delphi method
   - Interview
   - Focus group
   - Participant observation
   - Documentary analysis.

   Questionnaire:

   Advantage – large sample size and quick to administer to staff

   Disadvantages – difficult to develop one that would be suitable for elderly patients in hospital; respondents may answer what they want to say rather than what is really happening; may get poor response rate

   Delphi method:

   Advantage – likely to be well informed responses from a small number of respondents

   Disadvantage – based on current 'experts' knowledge and opinions on dietary supplementation, so may not create new knowledge

   Interview:

   Advantage – you can get in-depth understanding of dietitians', nurses' and patients' views on dietary supplementation and the underlying issues

   Disadvantages: time consuming and only likely to be a small sample size, so not generalisable

   Focus group:

   Advantage – a dietetic team viewpoint on dietary supplementation in the elderly could be gained in a reasonably small time frame

Disadvantage – the findings could be biased by the strong opinions of one focus group member

Participant observation:

Advantage – get a 'truer' picture of what is happening regarding dietary supplementation with elderly patients in hospital

Disadvantage – only likely to see dietary decision-making with a small number of patients

Documentary analysis:

Advantage – able to access a large quantity of data, e.g. dietitian and nursing notes, patients' case notes

Disadvantage – records may not be fully complete, and the process could be very time-consuming; will be unable to go back and clarify issues

3. **What is meant by the term 'triangulation' in relation to research design?**

Using more than one research method in an attempt to counteract the potential weaknesses of each. Triangulation should therefore produce more reliable findings.

Chapter 11

1. **What are the main ethical duties that should be considered before undertaking a research project?**
   a) protection of rights
   b) protection from harm
   c) positive contribution
   d) honesty and integrity.

2. **If you were undertaking a student research project involving interviewing clinical staff from which groups should you seek ethical approval?**

The manager in charge of the clinical area in question, the local Research Ethics Committee and the approval of the education institute.

3. **List the main headings required in a research proposal.**

Project title

Names, details, experience and qualifications of the researcher (this includes the researcher supervisor if this is a student application)

Research objectives

Outline of the research design

Scientific background to the study

Recruitment and sample details

Tests, tools, devices and drugs to be used

GP consent if required

Precautions to protect participants against potential discomfort, risk, breeches of confidentiality or the Data Protection Act

Informed consent process (including consent forms, and information sheets)

Indemnity forms if drugs or equipment are to be used

Likely costs and any sponsorship details.

Chapter 12

1. **When do you code data ready for analysis?**

Once it has been collated, before it is analysed.

2. **What sorts of basic descriptive statistical techniques can be applied to quantitative data?**

Frequency distributions, mean median and mode data and standard deviations.

3. **How does a researcher prepare qualitative data for analysis?**

By transcribing and presenting it as a written document. Quotes or sections that illustrate key themes and patterns may then be highlighted and coded.

4. **How are quantitative findings usually presented?**

In statistical and graphical formats and supplemented by explanatory text.

Chapter 13

1. **What are the main sections that should be contained in a research report?**

Title, abstract, introduction, method, findings, discussion and conclusions, recommendations, references, appendices.

2. **Identify three possible 'dangers' in writing up a research report.**

Do not underestimate the time and effort required for writing up a report – it will take up about one third of the total time spent on the research.

Do not overestimate the readers' background knowledge of your topic.

Do not use long, rambling sentences or explanations. Write simply and clearly.

Do not use too many 'I' statements. Focus on the topic and the data.

Do not pad out your report with irrelevant information or pictures.

Keep to the word limit if the research is part of a course of study.

3. **Through what routes can the findings from a research study be disseminated?**

Summaries of key points circulated locally

Conferences – presentations, seminars and posters

Research workshops

Local and national journal publications.

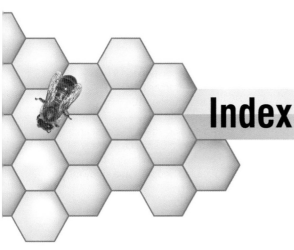

Index